W9-DFH-959

A Man's Guide to
Muscle
and
Strength

Stephen Cabral

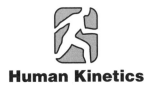

Human Kinetics

Library of Congress Cataloging-in-Publication Data

Cabral, Stephen, 1978-
  A man's guide to muscle and strength / Stephen Cabral.
    p. cm.
  ISBN-13: 978-1-4504-0220-0 (soft cover)
  ISBN-10: 1-4504-0220-8 (soft cover)
  1. Bodybuilding. 2. Muscle strength. 3. Physical fitness. 4. Men--
Physiology. I. Title.
  GV546.5.C34 2011
  613.713--dc23
                                    2011021475
  ISBN-10: 1-4504-0220-8 (print)
  ISBN-13: 978-1-4504-0220-0 (print)

This publication is written and published to provide accurate and authoritative information relevant to the subject matter presented. It is published and sold with the understanding that the author and publisher are not engaged in rendering legal, medical, or other professional services by reason of their authorship or publication of this work. If medical or other expert assistance is required, the services of a competent professional person should be sought.

The web addresses cited in this text were current as of August 2011, unless otherwise noted.

Acquisitions Editor: Justin Klug; **Developmental Editor:** Anne Hall; **Assistant Editor:** Tyler Wolpert; **Copyeditor:** Bob Replinger; **Permissions Manager:** Martha Gullo; **Graphic Designer:** Joe Buck; **Graphic Artist:** Kim McFarland; **Cover Designer:** Keith Blomberg; **Photographer (cover):** © Corbis RF/age fotostock; **Photographer (interior):** Neil Bernstein; **Visual Production Assistant:** Joyce Brumfield; **Photo Production Manager:** Jason Allen; **Art Manager:** Kelly Hendren; **Associate Art Manager:** Alan L. Wilborn; **Illustrations:** © Human Kinetics, unless otherwise noted; **Printer:** McNaughton & Gunn

Human Kinetics books are available at special discounts for bulk purchase. Special editions or book excerpts can also be created to specification. For details, contact the Special Sales Manager at Human Kinetics.

Printed in the United States of America   10 9 8 7 6 5 4 3 2 1

The paper in this book is certified under a sustainable forestry program.

Human Kinetics
Website: www.HumanKinetics.com

United States: Human Kinetics
P.O. Box 5076
Champaign, IL 61825-5076
800-747-4457
e-mail: humank@hkusa.com

Canada: Human Kinetics
475 Devonshire Road Unit 100
Windsor, ON N8Y 2L5
800-465-7301 (in Canada only)
e-mail: info@hkcanada.com

Europe: Human Kinetics
107 Bradford Road
Stanningley
Leeds LS28 6AT, United Kingdom
+44 (0) 113 255 5665
e-mail: hk@hkeurope.com

Australia: Human Kinetics
57A Price Avenue
Lower Mitcham, South Australia 5062
08 8372 0999
e-mail: info@hkaustralia.com

New Zealand: Human Kinetics
P.O. Box 80
Torrens Park, South Australia 5062
0800 222 062
e-mail: info@hknewzealand.com

E5307

A Man's Guide to

Muscle
and
Strength

Contents

Exercise Finder   vii   Introduction   xv

1 The Top 10 Training Principles to Lift By 1

2 Eat Right and Train Hard 11

3 The Death of Cardio as You Know It 23

4 Getting Started Is Easy 33

5 Starter Program 1 53

6 Starter Program 2 79

7 Pure Strength Workout 105

8 Core Power Workout 125

9 Strength and Power Workout 149

10 Hard Gainer's Workout 169

11 Functional Training Workout 191

12 Upper-Body Blast Workout 217

13 Hardcore Body-Weight Training Workout 241

14 The Road Ahead 267

References   269   About the Author   270

Exercise Finder

Follow this exercise index for quick reference to the exercises and equipment you'll need as you follow your own workout program.

Exercise	Equipment used	Page
Chapter 5: Starter Program 1		
Upper body		
Cable one-arm horizontal chest presses	Cable, 1 handle	60
Cable one-arm horizontal rows	Cable, 1 handle	63
Dumbbell two-arm shoulder presses	Dumbbells	66
Cable lat pull-downs in a squat	Cables, 2 handles	68
Cable EZ-bar triceps press-downs	Cable, EZ-bar	70
Dumbbell neutral to supinated curls	Dumbbells	71
Dumbbell ball chest presses	Dumbbells, stability ball	72
Dumbbell one-arm bent-over rows	Dumbbell	75
Lower body		
Backward alternating lunges	Body weight	58
Squat to stands	Body weight	59
Dumbbell Romanian deadlifts	Dumbbells	61
Dumbbell box front squats	Dumbbells, box	64
Dynamic forward cone lunges	Body weight, cone	67
Dumbbell box deadlifts	Dumbbells, box	69
Dumbbell one-leg step-ups	Dumbbells, box	73
Dumbbell two-arm sumo deadlifts	Dumbbells	76
Core		
Planks	Body weight, mat	57
JC band horizontal chops	JC band	62
Static bridging	Body weight, mat	65
Reverse crunches	Body weight, mat	74
Supermans	Body weight, mat	77

(continued)

Exercise Finder, *continued*

Exercise	Equipment used	Page
Chapter 6: Starter Program 2		
Upper body		
Dumbbell one-arm empty cans	Dumbbell	85
Cable two-arm horizontal chest presses	Cables, 2 handles	86
Cable two-arm horizontal rows	Cables, 2 handles	89
Chin-ups	Body weight, pull-up bar	93
Dips	Body weight, parallel bar dip handles	96
Dumbbell Zottman curls	Dumbbells	97
Declined push-ups	Body weight, bench	98
Dumbbell two-arm bent-over rows	Dumbbells	101
Lower body		
Lateral lunges	Body weight	84
Barbell back squats	Barbell	87
Dumbbell walking lunges	Dumbbells	90
Dumbbell one-leg Romanian deadlifts	Dumbbells	95
Dumbbell shoulder-loaded step-ups	Dumbbells, box	99
Upper body and lower body		
Dumbbell squat presses	Dumbbells	92
Upper body, lower body, and core		
Mountain climbers	Body weight	83
Dumbbell overhead squats	Dumbbells	102
Core		
Cable low to high chops	Cable, 1 handle	88
Dynamic bridging	Body weight, mat	91
Dumbbell axe chops	Dumbbell	94
Bench leg lifts	Body weight, bench	100
Medicine ball side-to-side rotations	Medicine ball, pad	103
Chapter 7: Pure Strength Workout		
Upper body		
Dumbbell flat chest presses	Dumbbells, bench	112
Barbell bent-over rows	Barbell	114
Barbell military shoulder presses	Barbell	116
Pull-ups (weighted)	Body weight, weight plate, pull-up bar	118

Exercise	Equipment used	Page
Barbell incline chest presses	Barbell, bench	120
Cable seated rows	Cable, V-bar, row machine	122
Lower body		
Transverse plane lunges	Body weight	110
Barbell back squats	Barbell	113
Barbell Romanian deadlifts	Barbell	115
Dumbbell deadlifts with pronated grip	Dumbbells	117
Barbell split lunges	Barbell	119
Dumbbell one-leg step-ups	Dumbbells, box	121
Barbell front squats	Barbell	123
Upper body and lower body		
Split jacks	Body weight	109
Upper body and core		
Hand walkouts	Body weight	111
Chapter 8: Core Power Workout		
Lower body		
Curtsy lunges	Body weight	130
Upper body and core		
T-twist push-ups	Body weight	137
Dumbbell one-arm prone rows	Dumbbell, bench	140
Cable low to high rope chops	Cable, rope	143
Lower body and core		
Barbell front squats	Barbell	133
Barbell one-leg good mornings	Barbell	138
Upper body, lower body, and core		
Squat thrusts (burpees)	Body weight	129
Barbell push presses	Barbell	132
Dumbbell one-leg reach to rows	Dumbbell	134
Barbell overhead squats	Barbell	141
Dumbbell walking lunges with chop	Dumbbell	146
Core		
Planks with shoulder abduction	Body weight, mat	131
Barbell combat twists	Barbell, landmine (optional)	135
Cable kneeling rope chops	Cable, rope, pad	136
Stability ball roll-outs	Body weight, stability ball, pad	139

(continued)

Exercise Finder, *continued*

Exercise	Equipment used	Page
Unilateral bird dogs	Body weight, mat	142
Medicine ball slams	Medicine ball, pad	144
Side planks with reach under	Body weight, mat	145
Cobras	Body weight, mat	148
Chapter 9: Strength and Power Workout		
Upper body		
Plyometric box push-ups	Body weight, boxes	157
Barbell inverted pronated rows	Barbell, bench press station	158
Cable supinated lat pull-downs	Cable, lat bar, pad	162
Dumbbell floor chest presses	Dumbbells	164
Cable pronated wide-grip seated rows	Cable, lat bar, bench	166
Lower body		
Skips in place	Body weight	153
Speed skaters	Body weight	154
Plyometric box jumps	Body weight, box	156
Barbell backward lunges	Barbell	159
Alternate split lunge jumps	Body weight	161
Barbell deadlifts from boxes	Barbell, boxes	163
Barbell deep box squats	Barbell, box	165
Cable rope pull-throughs	Cable, rope	167
Upper body, lower body, and core		
Dumbbell one-arm snatches	Dumbbell	160
Core		
Plank get-ups	Body weight, mat	155
Cable alternating horizontal chops	Cable, 1 handle	168
Chapter 10: Hard Gainer's Workout		
Upper body		
Barbell incline chest presses	Barbell, bench press station	176
Barbell bent-over rows	Barbell	178
Barbell military shoulder presses	Barbell	180
Alternate grip pull-ups	Body weight, pull-up bar	182
Barbell shrugs	Barbell	183
Dumbbell lateral raises	Dumbbells	184
Cable two-arm horizontal chest presses	Cables, 2 handles	185

Exercise	Equipment used	Page
Dips	Body weight, parallel bar dip handles	187
Cable supinated seated rows	Cable, lat bar, bench	188
Barbell curls	Barbell	190
Lower body		
Barbell Romanian deadlifts	Barbell	177
Barbell box step-ups	Barbell, box	181
Dumbbell walking lunges	Dumbbells	189
Upper body, lower body, and core		
Spidermans	Body weight	173
Dumbbell Zercher squats	Dumbbell	186
Upper body and core		
Plank one-arm reach-outs	Body weight, mat	175
Lower body and core		
One-leg dynamic bridging	Body weight, mat	174
Barbell front squats	Barbell	179
Chapter 11: Functional Training Workout		
Upper body		
Barbell supinated inverted rows	Barbell, bench press station	214
Lower body		
Vertical frog jumps	Body weight	197
Dumbbell Zercher step-ups	Dumbbell, box	199
Dumbbell Bulgarian split squats	Dumbbells, box or bench	202
Dumbbell goblet squats	Dumbbell	206
Dumbbell one-arm deadlifts from floor	Dumbbell	212
Barbell shoulder-loaded walking lunges	Barbell	215
Upper body and core		
Inchworms	Body weight	195
Dumbbell renegade rows	Dumbbells	201
Cable push-pulls	Cables, 2 handles	204
Turkish half get-ups	Kettlebell, mat	207
Stability ball pikes	Stability ball	208
Lower body and core		
Stick overhead squats	Stick	196
Barbell overhead forward lunges	Barbell	205

(continued)

Exercise	Equipment used	Page
Upper body, lower body, and core		
Barbell one-arm squat presses	Barbell, landmine (optional)	198
Kettlebell alternating one-arm swings	Kettlebell	203
Kettlebell cleans, front squats, and presses	Kettlebells	210
Kettlebell two-arm swings	Kettlebell	216
Core		
Oblique twists (slams)	Medicine ball, pad	200
Stability ball back reverse extensions	Stability ball	209
Hanging knee-ups	Body weight, ab straps (optional), pull-up bar	213
Chapter 12: Upper-Body Blast Workout		
Upper body		
Kettlebell alternating shoulder presses	Kettlebells	224
Chin-ups	Body weight, pull-up bar	225
Dips	Body weight, parallel bar dip handles	227
Cable criss cross raises	Cables, 2 handles	228
Cable overhead rope triceps extensions	Cable, rope	229
Medicine ball push-ups	Medicine ball	230
Cable one-arm horizontal rows	Cable, 1 handle	231
Cable supinated triceps press-downs	Cable, EZ-bar	234
Cable supinated wide-grip biceps curls	Cable, EZ-bar	235
Dumbbell shrugs	Dumbbells	237
Cable close-grip triceps press-downs	Cable, V-bar	238
Dumbbell Zottman curls	Dumbbells	239
Lower body		
Backward lunge press-outs	Medicine ball	222
Upper body and lower body		
Dumbbell deadlifts to cheat hammer curls	Dumbbells	226
Dumbbell squat to standing reverse flys	Dumbbells	233
Upper body, lower body, and core		
Jumping jacks	Body weight	221
Barbell push presses	Barbell	236
Kettlebell double swings	Kettlebells	240
Core		
Medicine ball slams	Medicine ball, pad	223
Bench leg lifts to hip thrusts	Body weight, bench	232

Exercise	Equipment used	Page
Chapter 13: Hardcore Body-Weight Training Workout		
Upper body		
Chair dips	Body weight, chair	256
Lower body		
Transverse plane lunges	Body weight, bench	246
One-leg pistol squats	Body weight	249
Bulgarian split squats with two-arm raise	Body weight, bench	252
Alternating dynamic forward lunges	Body weight	255
Prisoner deep squats	Body weight, box	261
One-leg good mornings	Body weight	263
Upper body and core		
T-twist push-ups	Body weight	248
Inchworms	Body weight	254
Hindu push-ups	Body weight	260
Lower body and core		
One-leg dynamic bridging	Body weight, mat	259
Upper body, lower body, and core		
Jumping jacks	Body weight	245
Mountain climbers	Body weight	247
Squat thrusts (burpees)	Body weight	264
Core		
One-leg-up crunches	Body weight, mat	250
Side planks with reach under	Body weight, mat	251
Alternating supermans	Body weight, mat	253
Planks with shoulder abduction	Body weight, mat	257
Shin slap V-ups	Body weight, mat	258
Brazilian crunches	Body weight	262

Introduction

Bill has a problem.

It's cold this morning, and Bill's alarm clock sounds while it's still dark. He's desperately searching for that magic button he can smack so that he can settle back in for another five minutes of pillow time. After the alarm blares a second time, he debates hitting the snooze button again but decides that he can't put off the inevitable forever.

So, it's time to start his day.

Bill's been trying to eat healthier lately, but he still doesn't know what exactly *healthy* means. Some people say that whole-wheat cereal is OK, but others want you to stay on a strict diet of lean protein and vegetables. Bill decides that he's too pressed for time to figure it all out this morning, so he grabs a bowl of his favorite cereal and sits in front of the TV as he's planning what he has to do the rest of the day.

Bill's to-do list is lengthy, and unfortunately for him, he has plenty of time to stress about it on the commute to his desk job.

At work Bill tries to beat the deadlines of the workday while calling back clients and shifting his inbox items to his outbox. All the while, Bill is seated at his ergonomically incorrect desk setup, staring at a computer and wondering how in the world his back and legs got so stiff.

Now it's lunchtime.

At lunch Bill goes out with some of his work buddies. Although he tried to persuade them to choose a healthy alternative that day, all the guys wanted to go out to their usual lunch joint and grab a couple of slices of pizza and a soda. Bill has been doing some research lately and has realized that all that junk he's been eating is just a load of empty calories, which is translating into an ever-expanding waistline. But he's with his buddies, and he doesn't want to be "that guy" eating the salad, so he submits and orders his standard two slices of pepperoni and a can of soda.

A few hours have passed since Bill went to lunch, and he can't understand why he's feeling exhausted. What does he have to be tired from? he wonders. All he's been doing is sitting at a desk all day. Bill checks his watch and can't believe that it's only three o'clock.

At this point he's debating whether he'll even have the energy to do his stale, once-or-twice-a week workout later tonight. Currently, he's torn between the offer he got earlier through e-mail to go out with a few friends after work or to take his girlfriend, whom he hasn't seen all week, out to dinner. He realizes that if he chooses either option, his plan of heading to the gym straight from work won't happen.

On this particular day it doesn't really matter what he would have chosen because just before 5:30 rolls around his boss asks him whether he could stay a little later tonight to finish up a project that needs to go out to a client the next morning.

Bill had no idea when he made the commitment to get back into shape that juggling everything would be so difficult. He now thinks that work, family, friends, and other commitments are always foiling his attempts to stay in a consistent routine.

Bill knows that there has to be an easier way, but he feels overwhelmed and doesn't know where to turn for answers.

How is he supposed to figure out what to eat, when to work out, or what he should be doing when he's read so many conflicting articles and reports from all those so-called experts? Everywhere he looks there is a new study explaining the newest and greatest method to get in shape. He is confused and on the verge of just giving up.

All Bill wants is a straightforward program that will allow him to regain his strength, conditioning, and confidence. He also wants to sculpt a body that he can be proud of. When he wears a T-shirt and jeans he wants both guys and girls to notice that he's been working out and taking care of himself. He wants the strong arms and chest that result from training the right way. Bill isn't necessarily seeking to develop a massive bulky physique like the guys on the covers of the muscle magazines that he glances at in the bookstore. Instead, he wants the healthy, lean, and defined look like the cover models for *Men's Health*.

He also realizes that he's not a guy with a lot of time.

Bill needs a program to fit his busy life that does not require him to spend hours in the gym five or six days a week. He has commitments to his girlfriend, his buddies, his family, and work that he's not willing to give up.

Bill is at a crossroads right now. He knows that if he keeps going as he is, he'll continue to lose muscle, add body fat, and look like the out-of-shape guys he has always looked down on. He wants to take care of his body and can't stand the fact that his belly is now hanging over his pants when he sits down at his desk. He also realizes that his sitting down on the way to work, at work all day, and on the way home isn't exactly a recipe for staying lean and fit.

Bill is lost—searching for answers that will transform his body and his life.

His quest to find a training system that will help him get stronger, more defined, and increase his confidence in the process has turned up more dead ends and bad advice than it has answers.

Until now.

The story that I just recounted to you was and is real. Although this account was based on a personal client of mine who walked into my studio seven months ago, it bears striking similarities to the lives of hundreds of thousands of guys around the world.

As men, we all share some basic aspirations and wants.

We all want to look good at the beach and feel comfortable with our shirts off. We want our significant others to find us attractive. We realize that our bodies say a lot about who we are and how we take care of ourselves.

Unfortunately, most of us are short on time and heavy on the kinds of temptations that pull us away from developing and attaining our ideal bodies.

There is an answer, though, and it's something that I developed only after more than 12 years and 15,000 sessions with private clients.

After reviewing hundreds (if not thousands) of the previous workout programs of guys I had been training to increase strength and transform their bodies, I stumbled across a few specific similarities in the programs of the men who got the greatest results.

I realized that I was on to something, so I set out to put my theory to the test.

I also knew that this new and revolutionary form of program design had to be built for real guys who live in the real world. I had to account for busy schedules, low-energy days from lack of sleep, last-minute cancellations, and everything else that busy men have to deal with on a day-to-day and week-to-week basis.

I believe that you have enough to worry about and what you really want is a straightforward strength-training program designed for real guys that produces real results—plain and simple.

That's exactly what you are now holding in your hands.

After testing all the possible variables of what worked best, I knew that I had the winner. It was irrefutable and backed up by outstanding results from men just like you who trained with me both online and in my studio.

What I had developed was a three-day-a-week workout program that any guy could do. It didn't require hours in the gym (only 30 to 40 minutes three times a week) and it allowed the client to customize his off days to include additional at-home workouts or fat-burning intervals that he could do if he had extra time that week.

Best of all, it worked every time.

All the guys had to do was plug themselves into the step-by-step system. What they came out with was truly remarkable. I had men losing 5 pounds (2.2 kg) in their first week and doubling their strength and power within the first 12 weeks. To this day I continue to get floods of stories from men using this program about how they are losing the thickness in their waists and adding size and definition to their arms and chests within just a few weeks.

In addition, depending on your short-, mid-, and long-term goals, you can choose any of the six-week programs outlined in this book. Whether you want to increase power, strength, agility, muscle, athletic conditioning, or a combination of all of them, you have the ability to handpick your program from the eight uniquely formulated six-week workouts contained in this book.

I have spent more than a year writing and designing this manual to ensure that every detail was accounted for, and now my private clients' programs are yours.

For the next 12 months I will be your personal trainer and coach. You'll have me to keep you accountable through the exercise journal that I've laid out for you in this book. I went so far as to cut through all the media clutter and research and provide you with the top 10 training principles you need to lift by. I promise that this will be the most straightforward and powerful strength-training and body transformation program that you have ever followed.

It's the answer that you've been looking for.

I truly want you to succeed and develop the body of your dreams, something that you can be proud of, and to know that you've taken a big step in taking back your health and vitality. You deserve it, and there's never been a better time to start than right now.

I'm committed to your success.

CHAPTER 1

The Top 10 Training Principles to Lift By

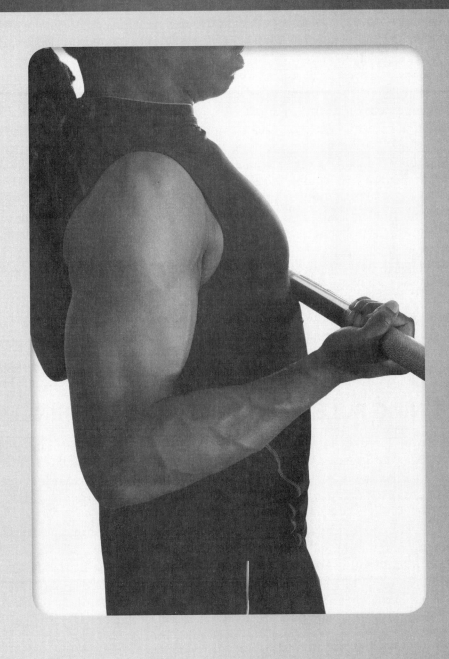

Wouldn't it be great if you could condense thousands of hours of exercise and training research on how to get the best results in the gym into just a couple of pages of cheat sheets?

I thought so, and I figured that others would, too, so I created this cheat sheet chapter about how you can use the most powerful training principles to transform your workout programs. This chapter will enable you to focus only on what matters most and free your mind of some of the less potent techniques that are nice but contribute only a small percentage of your total strength and physique gains.

This whole idea of cutting the clutter and digging deeper into what really makes the difference in getting results came from one of my strongest beliefs in life. It's called the Pareto principle, or Pareto analysis (often referred to as the 80–20 rule).

Basically, the rule states that 80 percent of your results or effects come from 20 percent of your actions or causes. Although this principle was originally used by the Italian economist, Vilfredo Pareto, concerning land distribution, it has far-reaching applications in every aspect of life, including your weight training. Many have theorized that as much as 90 percent of your results come from 10 percent of your actions (Koch 1999).

Because of this research, as well as my own training experience, I've whittled away 100 to 200 of the training rules and principles that you may have read about in magazines and online into a top 10 list.

Although it seems that a new article appears every day on the new best way to train, I can assure you that you need to incorporate into your program only a specific set of principles to see results.

In this chapter I've handpicked the Top 10 Training Principles to Lift By. If you follow these 10 principles and put them to work in your workout programs, I believe that your results will be nothing short of amazing. These principles have withstood the test of time and have been proven to work for all guys, whatever their genetic makeup.

My advice to you is to put on your information filter until you've firmly grasped the concepts of each one of these training principles. If you did nothing else but follow these top 10 principles, you'd have close to 90 percent of the skills that you need to advance your weight training. Of course, after you've mastered the techniques and knowledge from these 10, you can begin to branch out and expand your exercise education.

Now let's look at the Top 10 Training Principles to Lift By!

TRAINING RULE #1: FOLLOW THE SAID PRINCIPLE

SAID is an acronym for specific adaption to imposed demands. This phrase means that your muscles, energy systems, and nervous system will adapt to the training demands placed on them. Essentially, they will improve in all areas if the stimulus used is appropriate for what you are attempting to achieve (Baechle and Earle 2008).

In this book I will show you how you can use the SAID principle by safely increasing your weights each week. Eventually, you will plateau, and we will then change up your routine to keep getting results. This approach will promote greater hypertrophy in your muscles and huge improvements in strength and power. I've seen some of my clients put on slabs of muscle and dramatically increase their strength in a period of just 6 to 12 weeks by following this one training rule.

The key here is to keep pushing the bar higher each week by making small and steady improvements that over time add up to massive gains!

TRAINING RULE #2: IMPLEMENT EDT

Using Charles Staley's system of escalating density training (EDT), I want to show you how to increase your results by focusing on just one piece of this principle (Staley 2005). If you're not currently looking at how long your workouts are taking you, I recommend that you begin timing each workout routine. I want you to keep each workout to 45 minutes in length. We're going to cut out all the water cooler talk and 5-minute rest periods and get right down to business.

Building strength, power, and the body to match is a science. Fortunately, we now have the answers to unlock your potential. So from now on we're going to cut out any variables except how much weight you're lifting. Your reps, sets, rest periods, program duration, and all other variables will remain constant. Therefore, we will be able to unleash the SAID and EDT principles to complete more work in less time or the same amount of time.

TRAINING RULE #3:
MOVE IN MULTIPLE PLANES OF MOTION

The average exerciser never thinks about any movements other than those done in the sagittal plane (moving forward and backward). But by focusing on both the frontal plane (side-to-side movements) and transverse plane (rotational work), you will open up a completely new realm of possibilities for developing greater strength and becoming a more functional and well-rounded lifter.

Did you also know that you're likely to burn more calories and use more body fat by working in the frontal and transverse planes? The reason for this is that you're less likely to have made a neuromuscular adaptation to these movements, which means that your mind and nervous system will be trying to coordinate with your muscles on exactly how to complete these new exercises. Therefore, you will receive an added exercise boost!

In these upcoming programs I'm going to have you training like an athlete who can push, pull, and rotate with total control and power. This training rule will also allow you to develop and define muscles that you never knew existed on your body. (See figure 1.1 a and b on pages 4 and 5 for an illustration of the body's muscles.)

TRAINING RULE #4:
FOCUS ON MOVEMENTS, NOT MUSCLES

This principle is possibly the most overlooked rule in strength training. Most programs that men go through focus only on the muscle being worked. As a result, many guys choose exercises that leave their bodies misaligned, disproportionate, nonfunctional, stiff, and at risk for injury.

My goal is to help you to realize that by focusing on free-weight and cable-based exercises you will create a stronger, more functionally fit body. You'll quickly discover how much harder your body has to work when you're not seated in a stationary machine, which is one of the secrets to looking like an athlete. Remember, to look like a well-defined athlete you need to train like one.

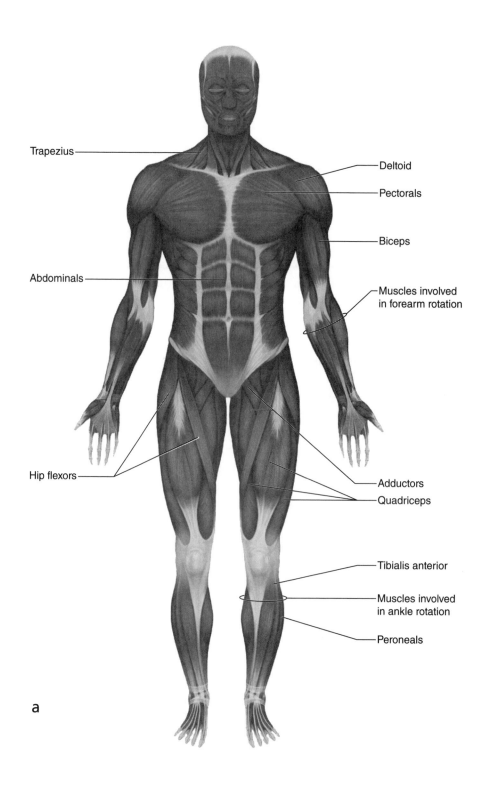

Trapezius

Deltoid

Pectorals

Biceps

Muscles involved in forearm rotation

Abdominals

Hip flexors

Adductors

Quadriceps

Tibialis anterior

Muscles involved in ankle rotation

Peroneals

a

Figure 1.1 *(a)* Front view of full body.

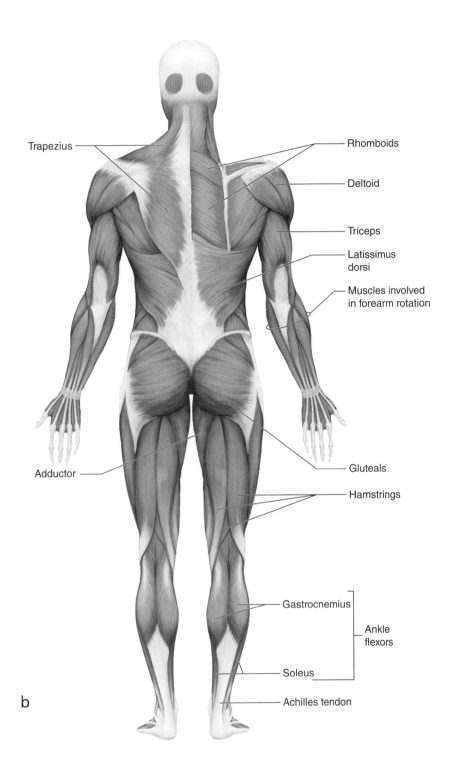

Trapezius

Rhomboids

Deltoid

Triceps

Latissimus dorsi

Muscles involved in forearm rotation

Gluteals

Hamstrings

Adductor

Gastrocnemius

Ankle flexors

Soleus

Achilles tendon

b

Figure 1.1 *(b)* Rear view of full body.

In addition, we're going to be using mainly compound, multijoint exercises that work more muscle groups to maximize your results. These compound lifts and movements—such as presses, pulls, rows, lunges, squats, deadlifts, step-ups, and chops—will allow you to attain the perfect proportional physique that not only looks good but also functions properly.

Although many of the exercises that I'm going to show you will have some new takes on old favorites, I assure you that you will not need a lot of equipment. I believe that you should be able to walk into any gym in the world and find the equipment that you need to get the job done. Using obscure workout devices only diminishes the likelihood that you will maintain consistency with your workouts, which is what strength training is all about.

I also need you to trust me that every workout will involve your core, abs, and arm muscles even if we're not directly targeting them with traditional crunches or curls. All of my male clients were worried at first that we weren't doing enough abdominal or arm work until they saw the results firsthand after just a few weeks of being on my program. Now they understand that the smaller muscle groups are working hard because they are blasting the larger muscles through compound movements.

TRAINING RULE #5: USE FULL ROM

Unless your physical therapist or doctor has advised you to use a limited range of motion, I highly suggest always working through a full range of motion (ROM) to maximize the degree to which the muscle fiber is being stressed and recruited during each movement. This technique will not only increase your muscle and strength gains but also allow you to remain strong through a full range of motion.

Remember the old saying "Use it or lose it." What that means is that you will literally get weak and unstable in your muscles and joints in the range of motion that you haven't been working. Men of all ages need to work through a full eccentric (the negative phase of the lift) and concentric (the positive phase of the lift) range of motion.

Even if you have to cut your resistance in half or use just your body weight, I suggest that you ease into this greater range of motion and incorporate this training rule into every one of your lifts. Your joints will become stronger and more stable, and your muscles will reveal new, untapped potential after they've become adapted to this new way of training.

TRAINING RULE #6: YOUR BODY CAN ONLY PUSH, PULL, AND TWIST

It's time to demystify the art of exercise program design. Let's start by recognizing that your body can work in only three ways. You can either push something, pull something, or rotate with your upper and lower body and your core.

We can further break down the exercise selections within your program to ensure that you perform push, pull, and rotational work within each workout to keep your body balanced and in proper alignment. And by using the right combination of supersets and tri-sets, you'll see how we can use these three motions to our advantage to get more work done in less time.

For example, you'll notice in many of the programs that I superset an upper-body pushing or pulling movement with its opposite lower-body countermovement. So, by choosing two compound opposing movements for the upper and lower body, we can work every muscle in the entire body! This is an amazing feat, and when you fully appreciate this technique you'll be able to cut your workout time while getting better results.

Also, your rotational work can include movements like planks and nonrotational torso chops that work your core by resisting rotation. We will explore this fairly new concept in this book. By using this new technique you will be able to tighten and tone your core without having to do crunches or sit-ups.

TRAINING RULE #7: USE A FAST–SLOW COMBO

The tempo mystery has long confused men training in the gym. Some experts say that you should move the weight over one second, pause for one second, and then decelerate the weight for four seconds. Others believe that you should move the weight over five seconds and then decelerate the weight over five seconds.

So much confusion, so little time. I've experimented with all of them, and to be honest, all of them work. How is that possible? The reason is that all approaches are means to the same end; all use a little known principle called time under tension. Because time under tension literally refers to how much time you're keeping your muscles under the tension of some type of resistance, you can see that your different tempos are all working to keep your muscle under tension for a specified period.

Although for some purposes, such as powerlifting, you may want to adhere to a slightly different set of guidelines, we're going to keep things simple and to the point in this book. Because our goal is to increase strength and develop a lean muscular body, we're going to use a tempo of 1-0-4 for most of our lifts (unless otherwise stated). This guideline means that when you are completing a chest press, you will push the weight quickly for one second, not pause at all at the top, and then lower the weight over approximately four seconds.

This method helps eliminate your stretch reflex, which allows your muscles to do less work because your tendons act like an elastic band to slingshot the weights back to their starting position. Studies show that by lowering a weight over four seconds during the eccentric phase of a movement, you eliminate most of the stretch reflex tendency, allowing more muscle fiber to be placed under tension, creating more muscle breakdown, and thus producing greater muscle growth as the fibers rebuild. The other big benefit to lowering the weight slower is that you eliminate any use of momentum, which only cheats your body out of getting greater results.

TRAINING RULE #8: LIFT WITH YOUR LEGS

Repeat after me: Running or doing cardio does not work your legs!

Aerobic-based work targets your cardiovascular system, namely your heart and lungs. This makes sense because the first thing to give out typically isn't your legs. Your cardio conditioning is what makes you stop.

Think about it another way: How many deep body-weight squats could you do before having to stop? Maybe you could do 50 in less than minute before your legs give out. When running, your legs can go for hours after you've conditioned your body, so after the initial adaptations have taken place during the first 6 to 12 weeks, your legs are not going to improve much with additional cardio. Therefore, to increase your leg size, strength, functionality, balance, alignment, and shape, you must train them with some type of resistance.

Also, endurance-based running (not sprinting) primarily targets Type I slow-twitch oxidative muscle fibers, whereas weight training goes after the more anaerobic Type II (a, x, and b) fast-twitch muscle fibers. These fast-twitch muscle fibers receive the most stimuli from short-duration exercises that force the muscles to generate near maximal force over a period lasting less than 30 to 90 seconds.

In addition, because over 60 percent of the muscle in your body lies between the top of your hip and your knee, you're severely limiting your metabolic response to your workouts if you aren't working those areas with some type of challenging resistance. This point is important because if you're not specifically targeting your glutes, quads, adductors, and hamstrings, you are missing a significant way of increasing your lean muscle and metabolism. You simply can't maximize your metabolism and fat-burning response from a workout if you're weight training only your upper body and doing cardio for legs. It just doesn't work that way.

TRAINING RULE #9:
USE ONLY ANABOLIC-BASED PROGRAMS

Men lifting three times a week should focus on major muscle groups, and preferably total-body training, with each workout. Unless you're in college or work in a gym, most guys simply can't get in a daily workout, which is completely understandable. You want working out to be part of your healthy lifestyle, not your entire life.

Three resistance workouts per week is plenty. This frequency will allow you to work every muscle in your body in each workout and incorporate different repetition ranges to ensure that you're maximizing your strength, power, and hypertrophy development. Another benefit to doing three full-body workouts per week is that your endocrine system will keep pumping out all-natural growth hormone and testosterone with each resistance day.

TRAINING RULE #10:
REST, RECOVER, AND REGENERATE

This rule is the forgotten principle in strength training. Most men see days off, stretching, and various types of massage as a waste of time or as something meant only for women. I can assure you that that this type of thinking will lead to countless overuse injuries to your joints and muscles, thereby sidelining you and keeping you out of the game.

In this book I will show you how to structure rest, recovery, and regeneration to lead to greater gains in all aspects of your lifting and life.

In addition, by using the "three Rs," I will let you in on the secrets to avoiding pain and injury, and instead enjoying a lifetime of benefits from strength training. We will review which stretches you should be doing, how many days you should be working out per week, when to take a week off, what nutritional approaches to recovery are best, and how you can use a self-massaging technique to decrease muscle soreness before it kicks in. And, in case all those benefits aren't enough, I'm going to show you how increasing your range of motion through stretching will improve your lifts in the gym!

I'll even fill you in on what some of the top Olympic and competitive athletes do to cut their recovery time in half while reenergizing their bodies.

By using the Top 10 Training Principles to Lift By, you will dramatically improve your chances for achieving your strength and muscle gain goals while keeping your body healthy.

You'll also find that the exercise selection, rest periods, and program design start to make a lot more sense in terms of why you're doing what you're doing. This point is important because many guys just go into the gym and repeat the same program that they've been doing for the past two years or, even worse, have no plan at all.

Having a set workout program that you can adhere to for four to six weeks should be the cornerstone for you and every guy who is putting in time at the gym. That's the reason I think that you'll find this book so useful. It will be your workout guide and virtual trainer to eight unique training programs, all built around your goal of developing a lean, toned, and defined body.

But having even the best workouts in the world won't get you the flat belly that you are looking for unless you follow the proper nutritional guidelines. In the next chapter I'm going to break down all the complex nutrition principles out there and provide you with a simple set of nutrition and nutrient guidelines that you can use to maximize your workouts.

OK, it's chow time, so let's talk about what you should be eating and when.

CHAPTER 2

Eat Right and Train Hard

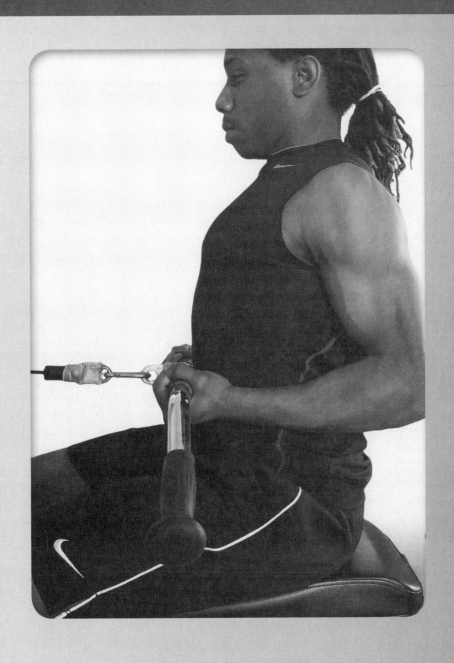

I hate it when people try to calculate how important nutrition is when it comes to building strength and muscle. Some people say it's 70 percent, some 80 percent, and others believe that it's half of the equation. I find those calculations arbitrary and close to useless.

Without a proper eating plan, you will struggle to get any of the results that you are looking for. No particular percentage pinpoints how important the right type of nutrition is to your weight-training results. In this regard you could say that it is 100 percent of the equation. You simply won't add size to your chest, arms, and legs without fueling your body with the right nutrients and sufficient calories to make the gains.

The great part about this is that following a nutritional plan that will produce noticeable results is not difficult. If you are willing to do a little planning, you'll see that the sample meal plans I have laid out for you may not be much different from how you are eating now.

Because entire books are devoted to nutrient timing, supplements, protein requirements, meal spacing, inflammatory response, and so forth, we'll look only at the most important elements that you need to follow to develop the lean, muscular physique that you're aiming for. As I said earlier, I believe that 20 percent of the details can produce 80 percent of the results. If you can focus on that, then you'll be way ahead of the game.

So let's get right to it.

Here are the main principles that you should follow if you don't want your hours in the gym to go to waste.

WATER

Whether your goals are to gain weight, get ripped, or just maintain a healthy physique, one staple that never changes is the amount of water that you need to consume on a daily basis. I know that we all have our good days when we drink plenty of water, but making sure that you're staying hydrated is of the utmost importance. First, if you're even slightly dehydrated you're going to begin to feel sluggish and rundown. In this situation you may go for a caffeinated pick-me-up to bring your energy levels back up, although you could possibly dehydrate yourself further if you are not a regular caffeine consumer. But before you reach for a coffee or Red Bull, drink at least 16 ounces (473 ml) of water and then wait to see whether that does the trick.

Second, you need to keep in mind that your muscles are about 70 percent water. If you're looking for fuller, thicker, more volumized muscles, you're going to need to replenish them with good old H_2O. Also, remember that fruit is predominantly water, so you can increase your hydration levels by eating vegetables and healthy dairy products.

You can throw out the old rule about drinking eight glasses of water a day. Instead, aim to consume 0.5 ounces per pound (15 ml per kg) of body weight per day. If you tip the scales at 180 pounds (82 kg), you'll want to drink close to 11 8-ounce (237 ml) glasses of water. Of course, your exact water requirements may be different. During the warmer months or if you're sweating a lot, you will want to consume more water, whereas during the colder months your hydration needs may be less. For a true test of your hydration levels look at your urine the next time you use the bathroom. If it's clear, you've had more than enough water; if it's the color of tea, you need to rehydrate. What you're looking for is a very light shade of yellow. At that point you will know that you are fully hydrated. (Keep in mind that some vitamins and foods affect the color of your urine, so you will need to wait until they have passed before calculating your true hydration levels.)

PROTEIN

Instead of trying to estimate your lean body mass (your weight minus your body fat) and then multiplying that by a number that seems to vary with each passing year, it's far easier to use this formula.

I've been having my private clients who want to add muscle take their body weight in pounds (or goal body weight) and aim for that many grams per day in protein. So if you weigh 180 pounds you should consume 180 grams of protein. (If you weigh yourself in kilograms, double your weight and add 10 percent to get your protein goal in grams.) Making sure that you're getting enough protein each day (even nonworkout days) is essential for several reasons. The main reason is that the protein and amino acids that you derive from them are the building blocks for muscle. Another reason is that protein is satiating and keeps your hunger level lower throughout the day.

The easiest way to take in your necessary protein requirements per day is by splitting the calculated amount over six or seven meals. For example, to reach 180 grams per day you could take in 35 grams of protein (only about 6 oz [170 g]) of lean meat) for breakfast, lunch, and dinner, which would give you 105 right off the bat. (Few meats, except turkey and a few others, contain as much as 7 grams of protein per ounce; most are 6 grams per ounce.) You could get another 60 to 80 grams by drinking two protein shakes during the day. In general, snacks like nuts or fruit are relatively low in protein, but they have other valuable nutrients, which is why you'll want to include a variety of foods in your diet. As you can see, this amount of protein may seem daunting at first, but it is easier to consume than you may think. Another point to keep in mind is that protein is thermogenic, which means that about 30 percent of all the calories that you get from protein are burned up in the energy required to digest those foods. You are less likely to get fat eating protein than you are by eating your typical pasta or cereal dishes!

GOOD FATS

I can't believe that fat still gets a bad rap. Let's straighten out one thing—fat does not make you fat. Eating a ton of calories consistently beyond your daily caloric needs from poor-quality foods, from any source (especially high-glycemic foods), is what makes you fat.

Good fat, like that found in oily fish, nuts, unprocessed oil, and avocado, is a powerful energy food. In addition, fat helps regulate your hormones naturally, allowing you to be the man you were meant to be. You'll have better-looking skin, hair, and nails, and you'll feel stronger and more powerful with that good fat in your diet.

You should consume higher dosages of omega-3 fatty acids because the typical U.S. diet is far higher in omega-6 fatty acids from saturated fat and processed foods. By taking in more omega-3 (or even a fish oil supplement) you will balance out your fat intake and greatly improve your health by decreasing your risk for inflammatory conditions (think auto-immune disorders, heart disease, high blood pressure, high cholesterol, arthritis, allergic responses, diabetes, and many others). You'll want to work on decreasing your omega-6 intake while increasing your consumption of omega-3 fatty acids. Although omega-6 fatty acids are necessary for good health, when they become unbalanced in relation to omega-3 fatty acids, you'll have higher levels of inflammatory markers within your body, leading to poorer health and vitality.

The only caveat to eating fat is that it contains 9 calories per gram, instead of 4 calories per gram as protein and carbohydrate do. This is nothing to be afraid of, but you want to be aware that eating a cup of walnuts may be a bit much. When snacking on nuts I recommend portioning out about a quarter cup, or one handful. Containing about 200 calories, this amount gives you an energy boost without weighing you down from high fat content. Also, always opt for raw, unsalted nuts like almonds, walnuts, or pecans. Roasted or pasteurized nuts lose much of their powerful antioxidant and nutrient-rich properties.

COMPLEX CARBOHYDRATES

Sometimes I feel as if I'm the only person willing to be the bad guy when talking about carbohydrates. But somebody has to do it, and it may as well be me.

You simply do not need to be eating whole grains all day long to be healthy. I'd even go so far as to say that you'd be unhealthy if most of your diet consisted of whole grains. Most whole grains have been so highly processed that they have little resemblance to the food that they started out as. Just think about it for a minute. How does the food that you buy in a bag or a box stay fresh for so long when it would go bad in less than half the time when cut in nature?

When choosing whole grains look for those that resemble what they looked like in nature. Whole-grain oatmeal, quinoa, millet, and amaranth are all great choices that even have a considerable amount of protein given that they are still predominantly a carbohydrate. Even some varieties of wheat can be healthy for people without gluten sensitivity as long as they have not been overprocessed or genetically modified.

Also, almost every whole grain is inflammatory. Inflammation is one of those words that you are going to hear a lot more of in the future when it comes to living longer and preventing disease. Remember, if you're creating inflammation from all the carcinogens that surround you in life and from stress, whether it is at work, at home, or from working out, you don't need to compound it by eating inflammatory foods. Inflammation within your body involves an increase in cortisol, which ends up breaking down your body from the inside out.

That's why I recommend that you get your carbohydrate from a far healthier food source that's easy to find in the grocery store. These carbohydrate-rich foods are the bright, colorful ones that line the refrigerated section. They're called vegetables.

I know, I know . . . vegetables. But you have to eat them to stay healthy, young, and fit. They provide powerful nutrients to help your body rebuild and regenerate between workout sessions, and they will help increase your fiber count. Consuming 38 grams of fiber (or more) per day is a good goal for staying healthy and trim. Also, don't limit the amount of vegetables that you consume with each meal (unless you get a stomachache) because eating more of the green variety of vegetables will help fill you up and feel satiated until your next feeding.

Fiber is vitally important to health and potentially even more important for men who are lifting weights and consuming extra protein. Eating fiber allows your body to pull toxins from your intestinal tract to be eliminated from your body. Fiber also prevents constipation and promotes proper colon shape (think less cramping and bloating).

Now let's talk about fruit. Again, I don't want to be the bad guy, but if you need to lose body fat, fruit isn't necessarily the best option for all-day munching. Excess body fat (especially around the waist) is a good sign that your insulin isn't regulating your blood sugar levels as well as it should be. Funneling more fruit sugar (fructose) into your blood isn't going to help the situation.

That's why I recommend eating your fruit for breakfast and after your workouts when your blood sugar may be lowest and when you can use that sugar spike to your advantage.

Besides veggies and fruit, sweet potatoes, yams, long-grain brown rice, lentils, dried beans and other legumes, chickpeas, quinoa, and a few other less-known healthy choices should be your staple carbohydrates. To be honest, unless you're an ectomorph (naturally very thin) I'd save the starchy carbohydrate like bread and pasta for your reward meals.

WHEN AND HOW MUCH TO EAT

Unless you're training to be a sumo wrestler, you're not going to want to follow the approach of eating one big meal per day.

Ideally, most men who are looking to get or stay lean and weigh around 180 to 200 pounds (82 to 91 kg) will shoot for about 400 to 500 calories per meal, take in about 200 to 300 calories per snack, and consume pre- and postworkout shakes. Of course, if you are active during the day or looking to pack on a lot of size, you'll want to increase your daily caloric intake.

If you want to get more scientific with your approach to eating, I highly recommend keeping a food journal and writing down exactly how many calories you consume each day. Breaking down the meals and foods into protein, carbohydrate, and fat will be even more helpful. After calculating how many calories you consume in an average week, you can recalibrate your plan by tweaking your calorie consumption. If you're looking to lose body fat I suggest decreasing your calorie consumption by about 20 percent, or 500 calories, per day (to lose 1 pound [.45 kg] per week). Another point to keep in mind is that you'll want to increase your protein intake while decreasing your overall carbohydrate intake if your protein intake is not in line with daily average requirements.

If you're looking to gain weight, you'll simply add 20 percent to your daily caloric consumption, or about 500 calories per day. If you're truly a hard gainer you'll want to ramp up your complex carbohydrate intake to keep up with your energy expenditure.

In both examples, a 500-calorie surplus or deficit was used because adding or subtracting 500 calories per day, or 3,500 calories per week, from your diet is what is needed to gain or lose 1 pound (.45 kg) per week. Of course, you can do this by altering your exercise program (duration or intensity), by taking in more or less calories, or by doing both.

Also, to allow your body to process the meal that you just ate before your next feeding, you need to wait about three or four hours, depending on the size of the meal and your activity level. If you just trained you can have a protein shake before and after your workout and then another meal about an hour after that. Your body is primed and ready to metabolize the fuel that you're giving it within the three-hour window surrounding your workout.

SUPPLEMENTS

Supplements are not as bad as many so-called health experts make them out to be. The unscrupulous corporations that lie about certain products in their marketing, on the other hand, should cause us to view the entire industry with extreme caution.

Repeat after me: "I do *not* need to be the guinea pig for testing new supplements that come to the market, no matter how much data the advertiser presents."

Repeating that mantra to yourself over and over will, I hope, keep you safe from products that could be potentially harmful to you. I personally believe that there are only a handful of supplements that you should consider taking. And, of course, all recommendations are strictly optional because you can get all the nutrition you need through whole foods. In any case, it's best to make your own informed decisions.

I will say, though, that many people have no issue with devouring a pint of ice cream or eating a doughnut, but for some reason they have a problem with using a completely natural whey protein. That seems a little backward because the high-fructose corn syrup, preservatives, artificial sweeteners, and rancid oils that are contained within many fast foods and treats are far more harmful to your body than a little extra vitamin C.

In addition, having a few supplements around allows you to make better relative choices when you're traveling, on the go, or need a high-quality quick food.

So, without further ado, here are my top supplement picks:

1. **Whey protein powder**: Sure, there's a lot of talk about casein as a slow-digesting protein powder, but to be honest many people who are lactose intolerant have a difficult time digesting it without getting bloating and gas. I stick with high-quality whey protein powder, and when I want to slow the digestion of the shake (like before bed), I just add some almond butter, coconut, or some other type of fiber or fat to the shake. Also, casein is a lower-quality milk product that is cheaper to make and less bioavailable than whey protein, meaning that you won't absorb nearly as much as its counterpart, whey protein. To me, there is simply no easier or quicker "whey" (sorry, I just had to) to give my muscles complete, perfect protein after my workout to begin the rebuilding process. In addition, getting your 150 to 200 grams or so of protein per day is far easier when you can drink some of them.

2. **EPA and DHA omega-3 fish oil**: No, you will not smell like fish. The Carlson Lemon fish oil is superb and will help balance out your omega fatty acids each day. Besides eating lots of vegetables, consuming fish oil is one of the easiest ways to decrease inflammation and increase energy levels. You can even use this oil as a salad dressing. If you're not big on taking one to three teaspoons (or one tablespoon) per day, then I suggest going with high-quality krill oil. Krill oil caps are much smaller than fish oil capsules, and you can take less because more is absorbed. In general, at least one gram of EPA and DHA is recommended per day to provide the full benefits of these powerful omega-3 oils.

3. **All the rest**: I could probably try to push the benefits of 12 other supplements that I really like, such as additional branch chain amino acids (BCAA), turmeric, ZMA, B-complex, greens and fruit powder, vitamin D3, a strong daily multivitamin, psyllium husk fiber, flax seeds, alkaline teas, creatine (for weight and muscle gain), glutamine, and a few others, but if you focus on creating a healthy daily food plan that includes lean protein, lots of vegetables, and a few fruits like berries, you'll be all set.

After fine-tuning your nutrition and maintaining a consistent eating plan for three to six months, you can look into adding additional supplements. I would try to maximize your gains with as little supplementation as possible at first (besides proper nutritional intake from whole foods) and then add a supplement or two at a time. This approach will allow you to see how the supplement reacts within your body and whether you are really benefiting from taking it. My last piece of advice is to research each supplement thoroughly before you take it. Make sure that it comes from a natural source whenever possible and that it has been on the market in that particular form for at least five years. Look through the independent research, data, and studies to see what effects it will have on your body.

YOUR NUTRITION CHEAT SHEET

I've briefly outlined the following 10 cheat sheet items for you to focus on. As I stated earlier, nutrition and supplementation is a huge subject to cover, but I want to leave you with some pointers that will help you achieve the body that you want without having to earn a master's degree in nutrition. I think that you'll find these tips easy to remember and easy to implement on your path to transforming your physique.

Careful With the Caffeine

Limit caffeine to breakfast or before your workout and keep it under 300 milligrams total per day or cut it completely out of your diet. Because coffee is acidic, I also recommend choosing green tea instead.

Fuel Up on Water

Drink at least .5 ounces per pound (30 ml per kg) of body weight, or about 3 liters of water per day, depending on your body weight

Use Cheat Meals to Your Advantage

Cheat meals, or reward meals, consist of foods that typically aren't part of your healthy diet plan. Most of my clients' cheat meals consist of pasta, fried foods, or maybe a few alcoholic drinks. The foods are usually starchy carbohydrates or simple sugars that you've been trying to eliminate from your daily intake. After the first 21 days of faithfully sticking to your healthy eating plan, shoot for 1 or 2 cheat meals a week spaced at least 3 days apart. Another way to look at it is to have a cheat meal every 10th meal (if you've already reached your goal weight). If you're still trying to drop some body fat aim for one cheat meal per week, which should help to restore leptin levels and keep you losing weight. Leptin is one of the hormones responsible for signaling your brain that you are full and that it does not need to continue storing fat.

Be Carbohydrate Conscious

Unless you're an ectomorph who is trying to put on a lot of size, strive to get most of your carbohydrates from fruits and vegetables. Although you should limit fruits until you reach your goal weight (or at least for the first three weeks when you are cleaning up your diet), you should add them back in to your diet, especially after your workouts. Postworkout fruit consumption will probably not be stored as fat because your body will be craving the phytonutrients from the fruit as well as the added sugar. If you're in a pinch and need to grab a sandwich for lunch, opt for a high-fiber wrap and just tear away as much of the bread or wrap as you can and toss it aside.

Watch the Dairy

If you have an allergy or find that dairy products cause you to get a little congested after you eat it, you may want to limit or eliminate dairy and milk products from your diet. Everyone should keep it to three or fewer servings per day of high-quality products that have undergone as little processing as possible. Dairy is a fantastic source of calcium, protein, and many other valuable vitamins, but if you're lactose intolerant you will want to find more digestible forms of dairy like low-sugar Greek yogurt or cottage cheese, two of my favorites. But if you cannot consume dairy because of a milk allergy or if you become congested from it, don't worry. You can get calcium from many other foods, such as green leafy vegetables.

Eat Your Fat

Remember, not all fat is created equal, and omega-3 fats are good for you. Include some olive oil, fish oil, flax oil, almonds, walnuts, avocado, or other good fats in your daily meal plan. They will have you feeling stronger, being more energetic, and looking younger!

Never Skip Breakfast

Studies have shown that if you eat breakfast you're more likely to lose body fat and stick to your nutrition plan. Moreover, you need that meal for many other reasons. Just think—you've gone the last 8 to 10 hours without any food, and if you wait until midmorning or so for lunch, you'll have gone more than half a day without eating. You'll be cramming all your calories into a half day, which isn't helpful for either your metabolism or your waistline.

Do This First Thing in the Morning

One of the best things you can do after not drinking any fluids for over eight hours is to have a 16-ounce (473 ml) glass of water. That only makes sense, right? That's why I suggest it be the first thing you do every morning. You'll earn bonus points if you drink it at room temperature and squeeze some fresh lemon in it to create a more alkaline (less acidic) environment in your body. Lemon is naturally alkaline, so it cuts the acidity in your body first thing in the morning.

Increase Fiber Intake

Consume 38 grams or more per day from vegetables, fruits, and unprocessed whole grains. You can use a psyllium husk supplement if necessary to increase your fiber intake.

You Literally Are What You Eat

How you feel and how you're aging is based largely on what you eat throughout the day. Your body is literally made up of the foods that you consume, so if you're consistently downing caffeinated beverages and starchy carbohydrate, then you can expect to see your pants size grow and your energy levels drop. On the other hand, if you're eating lively foods like vegetables, berries, nuts, good fats, beans, and lean protein, you'll look and feel amazing!

WEIGHT GAIN SAMPLE MEAL PLAN

Ectomorphs or anyone looking to put on serious size can work with this sample layout and daily meal plan:

7:00 a.m.: Breakfast

Spinach egg omelet (two or three whole eggs or three whites and one whole egg)

Spinach and mushrooms sautéed in olive oil over medium heat

Whole oatmeal with flax

Bowl of mixed berries

10:00 a.m.: Midmorning snack

1/3 cup of almonds or walnuts

Hummus and vegetables

12:30 p.m.: Lunch

Grilled chicken breast

Black beans or lentils

Sweet potato

Mixed greens salad with olive or flax oil and lemon

3:30 p.m.: Midafternoon snack

Greek or Icelandic plain yogurt with almond slivers

5:00 p.m.: Preworkout shake *(consumed 30 minutes before your workout, only on workout days)*

Protein shake (30–40 grams of whey or vegetarian protein powder)

One piece of fruit

12–16 ounces (355–473 ml) of water

5:30 p.m.: Workout

30–45 minutes of training

6:30 p.m.: Postworkout shake *(consumed immediately following your workout, only on workout days)*

Protein shake (30–40 grams of whey or vegetarian protein powder)

One piece of fruit

12–16 ounces (355–473 ml) of water

7:30 p.m.: Dinner

Grilled salmon (drizzled in olive oil and lemon)

Brown rice

Broccoli or another colorful vegetable

10:00 p.m.: Pre-bed shake

Blended protein shake with almond butter

STAY LEAN AND ADD MUSCLE SAMPLE MEAL PLAN

Mesomorphs or anyone looking to stay lean while trying to add muscle should work with this sample layout and daily meal plan:

7:00 a.m.: Breakfast

Spinach egg omelet (two or three whole eggs or three whites and one whole egg)

Spinach and mushrooms sautéed in olive oil on medium heat

Bowl of mixed berries

Coffee or tea (optional)

10:00 a.m.: Midmorning snack

1/4 cup of almonds or walnuts

Hummus and vegetables

12:30 p.m.: Lunch

Grilled chicken breast

Black beans or lentils

Mixed greens salad with 1 tbsp olive oil or flax oil and lemon

3:30 p.m.: Midafternoon snack

Greek or Icelandic plain yogurt with almond slivers

5:00 p.m.: Preworkout shake *(consumed 30 minutes before your workout, only on workout days)*

Protein shake (30–40 grams of whey or vegetarian protein powder)

One piece of fruit

12–16 ounces (355–473 ml) of water

5:30 p.m.: Workout

30–45 minutes of training

6:30 p.m.: Postworkout shake *(consumed immediately following your workout, only on workout days)*

Protein shake (30-40 grams of whey or vegetarian protein powder)

One piece of fruit

12–16 ounces (355–473 ml) of water

7:30 p.m.: Dinner

Grilled salmon (drizzled in olive oil and lemon)

Broccoli or another green or colorful vegetable

10:00 p.m.: Pre-bed shake *(optional)*

Blended protein shake with almond butter

LOSE FAT AND ADD MUSCLE SAMPLE MEAL PLAN

Endomorphs or anyone looking to lose body fat while trying to add muscle should work with this sample layout and daily meal plan:

7:00 a.m.: Breakfast

Spinach egg omelet (two or three whole eggs or three whites and one whole egg)

Spinach and mushrooms sautéed in olive oil on medium heat

Coffee or tea (optional)

10:00 a.m.: Midmorning snack

1/4 cup of almonds or walnuts

Hummus and vegetables

12:30 p.m.: Lunch

Grilled chicken breast

Black beans or lentils (optional)

Mixed greens salad with 1 tbsp olive oil or flax oil and lemon

3:30 p.m.: Midafternoon snack

Greek or Icelandic plain yogurt

8 ounces (237 ml) of green or Yerba Mate tea (optional)

5:30 p.m.: Workout

30–45 minutes of training

6:30 p.m.: Postworkout shake *(consumed immediately following your workout, only on workout days)*

Protein shake (30-40 grams of whey or vegetarian protein powder)

One piece of fruit

12–16 ounces (355–473 ml) of water

7:30 p.m.: Dinner

Grilled salmon (cooked in olive oil)

Broccoli or another green or colorful vegetable

10:00 p.m.: Pre-bed snack *(optional)*

Cut up vegetables and hummus

CHAPTER 3

The Death of Cardio as You Know It

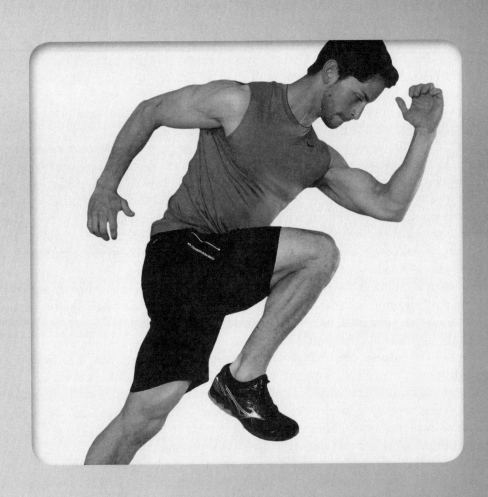

Unless you're training for an endurance-based sport, are concerned about doing traditional cardio for your heart, or just love the high that you get when you go out for a long run, you really have little need for long, slow, steady-state cardio. By steady state I mean that you are maintaining a consistent pace and heart rate for most of the cardio session.

Now, you may be thinking, what other kind of cardio is there? If you are, this chapter is going to be an eye opener. Even if you have an idea about what I'm going to share with you, I think you'll find this cutting-edge information enlightening.

This information is powerful because it means that any guy who would rather do laundry than go for a long run now has options! Those options all center on one fundamental type of training—high-intensity, interval-based training. At its essence interval training is spiking your heart rate for a short time and then allowing it to recover during a specified rest period.

Typically, the high-intensity part is a short-duration effort on a bike, elliptical machine, versa climber, or rowing machine; a body-weight exercise; a run; or any other approach that can blast your heart rate to about 90 percent of your max within 20 to 60 seconds. (To calculate your approximate maximum heart rate, just subtract your age from 220. That number represents 100 percent of your max.)

In a minute I will go into detail about how and why this type of training will revolutionize the way that you look at cardio and the way that interval training can transform your body. For now, though, I'd like to share with you a few reasons why steady-state cardio may be holding you back from reaching your peak potential. The two most important reasons are that cardio is self-limiting and that you end up getting fewer results from putting in more time.

Let's first talk about how you'll quickly outgrow your steady-state cardio program. As I said earlier, getting body transformation results from endurance-based aerobic cardio is self-limiting. You'll have to continue to run farther or faster to get better results (SAID principle). The reason for this is that your body is an extremely efficient machine that is the master of adaptation. In just four to six weeks after beginning any new routine, your body will adapt to the specific movements and intensity. It will lower its energy exertion to conserve calories, thus decreasing the effectiveness of your workout.

So when you look at it this way, how far are you willing to run or how much time do you really want to spend on a cardio machine? Is an hour and a half or two hours of cardio worth your time? Of course not. In addition, doing that much cardio can be catabolic, meaning that you'll lose muscle.

Yes, you heard that correctly. You'll actually begin to burn muscle with all that long-distance cardio. This happens when your body taps into your muscle reserves during longer workouts. It can also happen during times of high cortisol output, which happens during longer cardio sessions as well. Now, don't get me wrong. If you're in proper body alignment and are already in great shape, I'm not saying that running is bad for you or that it can't help you burn more body fat. What I'm saying is that it is neither the most efficient way to burn body fat nor the healthiest.

Let's also look at the speed factor. If you end up pushing yourself harder during your long-distance endurance cardio sessions, you will quickly hit a wall when your heart rate spikes too high, preventing you from maintaining that speed for your longer sessions. In addition, if your goal is to stay within your fat-burning zone, you're no longer tapping into as much of your fat stores as your cardio machine would lead you to believe. This brings me to another topic of discussion and one of the reasons why many people force themselves to do long, slow, boring cardio in the first place.

We've been led to believe that by staying in the fat-burning zone you will burn the greatest number of calories from fat compared with training at a higher or lower intensity. But nothing could be further from the truth. It's just one more strike against traditional cardio as you know it.

First, you burn the greatest percentage of calories from fat when you're spaced out in front of the TV or in bed sleeping. Now that doesn't mean that you're burning many calories, but nonetheless you are burning a greater percentage of calories from fat.

THE FAT-BURNING ZONE MYTH

As you may know, running at about 60 percent of your maximum heart rate will have you burning fewer calories than running at a higher intensity, but a higher percentage of those calories (about 50 percent) will come from fat. For that reason, doing cardio at 60 to 80 percent of your maximum heart rate is typically considered working in the fat-burning zone.

But this is where it gets good. If you keep your working sets (resistance exercises and sprints) at a higher intensity at around 85 percent of your maximum heart rate using interval-based training, you will burn more total calories, although a smaller percentage (about 40 percent) will come from fat.

Now if you were to glance at these stats you might think that doing cardio at a lower intensity would be the better choice to burn more fat, but closer inspection will show that, although high-intensity workouts burn a smaller percentage of fat, they actually burn more total fat. The reason for this is that the higher-intensity workouts burn more total calories, allowing a greater number of calories to be burned from fat even though the percentage is lower than in slower-paced cardio sessions. So even though you'll burn a smaller percentage of fat during your workout, you'll still end up burning more calories from fat in the end!

The foregoing argument doesn't mean that you should avoid doing any longer-distance aerobic cardio, because it can still be beneficial for endurance and cardiovascular health. But if body transformation or athletic performance is your main goal, I recommend following the high-intensity, interval-based programs that I will lay out for you in this book so that you can make steady progressions, thereby improving your strength-training and fat-burning results.

Another point to remember is that you can get the same interval-training effect, that is, spiking your heart rate and then allowing it to recover, by doing resistance-based workouts. Keep in mind when you're reading these upcoming programs that, unless I am doing my sprint triathlon training, I don't do a drop of traditional cardio, and neither do my private or online clients.

My private clients and I follow my specific style of programming that allows you to simulate cardiovascular training while simultaneously stimulating muscle growth and definition from fat loss. This environment is created by doing multiple compound movements back to back in superset or tri-set fashion, which results in greater time under tension without time for sufficient recovery between sets. After the superset, tri-set, or circuit is complete, you then rest 1 to 5 minutes depending on your program design. The intensity of moving challenging weights over the course of 90 to 120 seconds straight forces your heart rate to spike. As a result your body feels the aftershock effect of the interval that just took place.

This style of training is the best of both worlds, because your muscles are being worked to the max and your cardiovascular system is pumping much harder than it does when you go for a jog in the park. And you get them both done at the same time!

BURN FAT FOR UP TO 38 HOURS AFTER EACH WORKOUT

Did you know that by using the high-intensity interval principles just outlined you're going to get a greater fat-burning metabolic effect for up to 38 hours after each workout?

Multiple studies have shown an increase in metabolism for 31 to 38 hours after a high-intensity workout. This effect cannot be caused by steady-state cardio. Your workout must be intense enough for the body to have to work near maximum capacity (around 90 percent) during your interval sprints or working resistance sets.

Contrary to what many fitness experts say, this metabolic effect is not just about excess postexercise oxygen consumption (EPOC). Although it takes longer for your heart rate to recover after completing an interval-based workout versus a steady-state one, there is more going on here than just the EPOC effects.

According to a recent study in the *Journal of Applied Physiology and Occupational Physiology,* researchers at the Flinders University of South Australia believe that the elevated metabolic state that is created from near peak level training implies "that the EPOC is more than mere repayment of the O_2 deficit because metabolism is increasingly disturbed from resting levels as exercise intensity and duration increase due to other physiological factors occurring after the steady-state has been attained."

In my continuing research on this topic, I have also seen that engaging in a high-intensity workout program affects the mitochondria, blood sugar, insulin, leptin, enzymes, and many other hormonal and metabolic factors. What this means is that after your interval-based strength and sprint workouts you're going to metabolize sugars better without them being stored as fat. Also, you'll be far more likely to continue feeling the fat-burning effects for more than a day.

Additional research studies are finding that the duration of your workout is not necessarily a factor in lasting metabolic effects. More important is the intensity of the work performed. This is another reason why my 30- to 45-minute training sessions have worked so well for my online and studio clients!

Needless to say, the days of 60- to 120-minute workouts are over.

BURN 5 TO 10 PERCENT MORE FAT PER WORKOUT

Now before we get into what I'd like you to do on some of your non-weight-lifting days for interval sprints, I want to share with you one more tip on how to burn 5 to 10 percent more fat per workout. Who doesn't want to have a tighter waist with more well-defined abs?

A study performed by Jie Kang and the Human Performance Laboratory in Packer Hall showed that participants who started their cardio workouts slowly and then finished their routines (the second half) at a fast pace burned more calories.

When the researchers compared the results of the group who started out fast in the first half of the workout and then finished slower, they saw that the group of strong finishers burned 5 to 10 percent more fat per workout. In this particular study the researchers looked at fat burned through caloric expenditure, which they translated into stored fat burned. As we know, many variables determine whether the caloric expenditure will come from stored fat or from other energy sources, but in either case, the total energy expenditure was greater in the group that finished their cardio workouts at a faster pace.

So why I am telling you this?

Typically, when most guys begin an interval-based resistance or sprinting program, they ease into it and warm up their bodies safely before the big battle that awaits them. As they progress into the workout, the intensity becomes greater and they peak toward the 20- to 40-minute mark (based on the testosterone cortisol ratio). By using the programs that I've designed for you in this book, you're going to get the additional benefits of safely progressing up in weight while building intensity like a locomotive as you complete each additional set.

All this translates into muscle-swelling gains and powerful fat-burning effects! So now that you know exactly why interval training is so beneficial and much more potent than its counterpart—long, slow cardio—let's discuss one more point before we look at the exact intervals that I'd like you to follow.

WHICH CARDIO MACHINE IS BEST?

One of the most frequent questions I receive is this: "What is the best piece of cardio equipment to maximize calorie burn?" Now as we know, it's not all about calorie burn but rather the effects created during a short, high-intensity workout that carry over after your workout is done for the day. Regardless, I understand what the question is getting at, and I want to share the answer with you and put this debate to rest.

If you're looking strictly at which cardiovascular piece requires the most energy expenditure—elliptical, treadmill, rowing machine, or upright bike—then you will find that the answer lies in the amount of work that is asked of your body when using each piece. All other things being equal, the act of running requires your body to do more mechanical work, and thus the treadmill burns more calories than the others do.

Although ellipticals can provide a great workout, their smooth, comfortable motion works against them when it comes to forcing the body to absorb impact, resist rotation, and perform other actions that add up to increased caloric expenditure.

Here is a calorie comparison of the most-used gym cardio machines. The statistics are based on a 180-pound (82 kg) man moving at a moderate pace for 45 minutes. Your caloric expenditure may be smaller or greater depending on your age, weight, fitness level, or activity duration.

Elliptical—441 calories burned

Treadmill—675 calories burned

Rowing machine—476 calories burned

Upright bike—536 calories burned

You can see from the statistics that the treadmill outperformed all the others and the elliptical came in last. Again, the reason for this is simple. The exercise that forces the body to perform the greatest amount of biomechanical work will burn the most calories by engaging more muscle. Although I think that the calorie readouts on the screens of most cardio pieces at the gym are inflated, the numbers here give you a sense of where you'll get the most bang for your buck.

Personally, I prefer my clients to perform body-weight exercises like squat thrusts (burpees), jumping jacks, or mountain climbers because they can be done anywhere and are just as effective as using a cardio machine for interval work.

Of course, if you have access to a track, hill, or long stairwell, I highly recommend adding those high-intensity sprints as well.

Now that you know what you need to do to maximize your results in your training program, let's talk some specifics about how you're going to go about it.

As you'll learn in the following chapters, I've developed a realistic and proven system of strength training that you need to do only three times per week for maximum effectiveness. Although these three workouts would be enough training for the week on their own, I added some high-intensity, interval-based cardio work for anyone who wants to burn more fat or increase his athletic ability.

So, if you're following a Monday, Wednesday, and Friday weightlifting schedule, you should aim to include one or two of these sprint workouts per week. Remember not to train more than three days in a row to give your body adequate time to recover and regenerate.

Here are a few sample schedules that my clients have found beneficial. The first program is a consistent three days on, one day off, two days on, one day off, and repeat:

Three Resistance Workouts and Two Interval Sprint Days:

Monday: Resistance workout 1

Tuesday: Interval sprint day 1

Wednesday: Resistance workout 2

Thursday: Rest (three Rs)

Friday: Resistance workout 3

Saturday: Interval sprint day 2

Sunday: Rest (three Rs)

The next program is for men who need a little more time to recover between workouts or for those guys who are hard gainers in the gym. You'll work out every other day during the week and then choose one weekend day for your interval sprint day.

Three Resistance Workouts and One Interval Sprint Day:

Monday: Resistance workout 1

Tuesday: Rest (three Rs)

Wednesday: Resistance workout 2

Thursday: Rest (three Rs)

Friday: Resistance workout 3

Saturday: Interval sprint day 1 or rest

Sunday: Interval sprint day 1 or rest

You could add one of the high-intensity interval days to the end of one of your resistance workouts, but I suggest making it an abbreviated version and including it only during peak training periods.

So now that you know how to lay out your program, here are the interval sprint-training programs that you can add to your three resistance-training workouts per week.

You may complete any of these interval sprint workouts by using mountain climbers, squat thrusts, fast jumping jacks, running sprints, upright bike sprints, rowing, versa climber sprints, hill sprints, staircase runs, kettlebell swings, or any other high-intensity activity that will get your heart rate up to 90 percent of your maximum within the allotted time. If you do not have access to a heart rate monitor you should just think about using an all-out effort, because the only way that intervals work to boost your metabolism for an extended period is by creating a massive shock to your system from the high intensity. Keep in mind that if you do not need to rest when your sprint time ends, then your interval work set wasn't intense enough!

20-40 SPRINT WORKOUT

The 20-40 sprint workout is probably the best all-around sprint workout. It's fantastic for beginners because the 20 seconds of sprinting is not too long, and advanced exercisers don't have to pace themselves at all and can just go all out for the entire 20 seconds. Similar programs include 30-60 and 60-120 work-to-rest ratios, but until you've mastered the 20-40 sprint workout, you don't need to look into ramping up your sprint time. Just remember that when it's time to sprint for 20 seconds, you need to give an all-out effort. When the 20 seconds is up, stop your sprint and rest (without sitting) for 40 seconds before repeating.

Warm-Up: 5 Minutes

Warm up using one of the dynamic warm-ups included in this book or complete a general warm-up of the interval exercise that you are about to do at 50 percent of your intended pace.

Sprint Workout: 5 to 10 One-Minute Rounds

20-second sprint: 90 percent of max

40-second rest: Walk slowly around and do not sit or stand still

Using a 1:2 work-to-rest ratio, you will complete 5 to 10 rounds during which you sprint all out for 20 seconds nonstop. When the 20 seconds are up, you can walk around to catch your breath for the next 40 seconds. When your timer hits 1 minute, it's time to sprint as fast as you can again!

Repeat this 20-40 formula for as many rounds as you can (up to 10) with good form. (After a month or two you may choose to increase the 20 seconds of work to 30 seconds and the 40 seconds of rest to 60 seconds. The effort should still be all out, and the stimulus will be slightly different, giving your body a new challenge to adapt to.)

Cool-Down Recovery: 5 Minutes

After you have finished all your interval rounds, complete a 5-minute recovery by going for a light jog, walk, stair climb, or by performing body-weight exercises. This cool-down will allow you to recover safely by lowering your heart rate, flushing lactic acid, and lengthening your muscles.

Stretching: 5 to 10 minutes

I also recommend doing some foam rolling or static stretching directly after your recovery period (cool-down).

As you can see the whole program can be completed within just 20 to 30 minutes, and it will be far more effective in attaining your ideal body and health than those long, drawn-out, slow cardio sessions.

Here are two more interval sprint workouts that you can use along with the 20-40 sprint workout. (Use the same warm-up, cool-down recovery, and stretching as you did for the 20-40 sprint workout but substitute in any of these different work portions instead of the 20 seconds of work and 40 seconds of rest.)

Ladder Sprint Interval Workout

This fun workout is guaranteed not to be boring! Also, I like this sprint workout, because you can gradually ramp up to your maximum sprint about halfway through the workout. Another reason that the ladder sprint interval workout is a favorite is that your time is up before you know it. In just 12 minutes of full-throttle intensity, you will have blown through this interval workout. The ladder sprint interval workout is a great additional interval to add on your resistance-training days when you are trying to fine-tune your physique.

Sprint Workout: 11 Undulating Sprints

10-second sprint

10-second rest

20-second sprint

20-second rest

30-second sprint

30-second rest

40-second sprint

40-second rest

50-second sprint

50-second rest

60-second sprint

60-second rest

50-second sprint

50-second rest

40-second sprint

40-second rest

30-second sprint

30-second rest

20-second sprint

20-second rest

10-second sprint

10-second rest

Tabata Sprint Interval Workout

This interval was used as an experiment at the University of Fitness and Sports in Tokyo, Japan. Tests by Dr. Izumi Tabata and his colleagues revealed that their interval workout elevated fat-burning effects for up to 31 hours. The more impressive statistic was that the workout consisted of only 4 minutes of work on an upright bike! But don't let the short duration deceive you, because most people can't complete this extremely challenging interval on their first attempt. I recommend aiming for four of the eight rounds to start and working your way up by an additional round each week or when you feel ready. This is a great workout to do on the days when you have only 10 to 20 minutes, because all you have to do is fit in a quick 5-minute warm-up and you're ready to get cranking. Check out the Tabata sprint interval workout and remember that the 20 seconds has to be an all-out effort!

Sprint Workout: Eight Rounds of 20-10

20-second sprint (round 1)

10-second rest

20-second sprint (round 2)

10-second rest

20-second sprint (round 3)

10-second rest

20-second sprint (round 4)

10-second rest

20-second sprint (round 5)

10-second rest

20-second sprint (round 6)

10-second rest

20-second sprint (round 7)

10-second rest

20-second sprint (round 8)

10-second rest

I hope that you enjoyed this chapter about the death of cardio, and I'm sure that you're beginning to see that there is a science behind getting great results. The other good news is that developing a strong, lean, powerful physique does not require spending hours in the gym or slugging away on long, boring cardio sessions.

There is a better way, and we're just getting started!

Now it's time to move on to what this book really holds for you, which is the key to unlocking your peak potential (and even how to push past stubborn genetic plateaus). In the next chapter you're going to learn how to dive right into these eight, power-packed, six-week strength-training programs. After reading what these unique programs can do for you, I know that you're going to feel that renewed sense of motivation that you've been looking for!

CHAPTER 4

Getting Started Is Easy

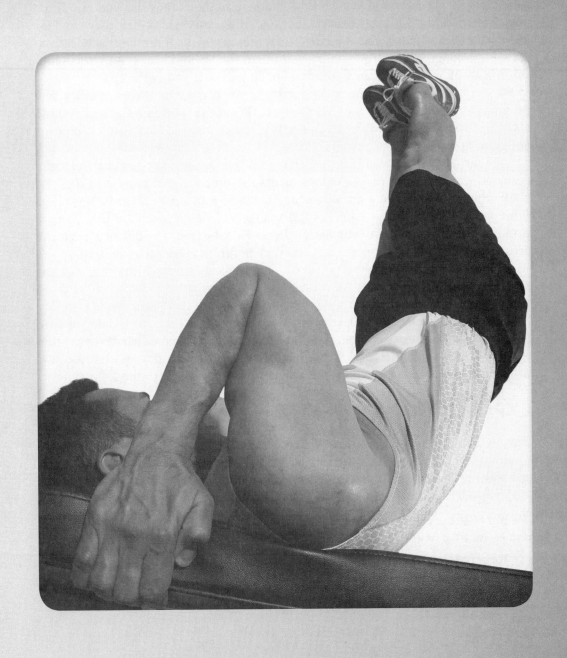

The best way to reach your goals faster than you could on your own is to find a step-by-step system that has been proven to work and then just plug yourself into it.

Whether I was training for my black belt in martial arts or competing in my first sprint triathlon, I looked to people who were more experienced in those fields and asked them to write up a plan that I could use to become successful. This is why I am excited for you to begin these new strength-training programs that I have designed for you.

I have been helping clients for over 14 years to get the bodies that they want and the strength and power to match. I can assure you that I have a plan that you can implement and begin to see results within a few short weeks, not months.

DON'T OVERCOMPLICATE THINGS

I want to warn you right now that your previous background, experience, and biases may prevent you from following the workouts exactly as they are laid out. This advice is important for a few reasons. For one, many guys think that they need far more volume (sets, reps, and exercises) than they really do. This approach leads to severe overtraining and produces less gain than they would like. I used to fall into this mind-set myself and can assure you that it will hurt you in the end.

For that reason among others, I suggest that you use the first week of every new program as an unloading week. This first week will ease you into the new routine and allow you to find the right weights to begin with and the ones you will eventually work up to.

Another reason that you want to stick with the plan is that it was specifically designed so that each workout complements the others. For example, if the first workout for the week had a horizontal pull like a one-arm row, then the second or third workout will have a vertical pull like a lat pull-down to ensure that you are working all the muscles in your back properly. I look to create balance in all my program designs, and therefore each six-week program is sufficient in itself.

A third reason that you don't want to overcomplicate things is that you can rest easy knowing that you're not the guinea pig for any of these workouts. These are tried, true, and proven to work. I handpicked the best of the best for you!

I will say, however, that I believe in staying active outside the gym and having fun. So if you want to go rock climbing, swimming, in-line skating, or whatever it is that you enjoy, then I say go for it. Just use it as one of your cardio days so that you stay within the framework of the program and do not become overtrained.

EXPLANATION OF TERMS

Throughout the book you'll see a few key terms and phrases that you need to know about up front. You may have seen some of them before, but I'd like to explain them in a way that we can all understand rather than in the typical textbook jargon.

Here's a list of key words that you will want to know:

• **Sets**: A set is simply the number of times that you complete an exercise. The set begins when you pick up the weight and ends when you put down the weight.

• **Repetitions** (**reps**): Reps are the number of times that you lift or contract and extend the muscle group that you are working. For example, for some sets you will move the weight only 3 times (3 reps), whereas for others you will perform 20 repetitions.

• **Tempo**: Tempo refers to the speed at which you move the weight (which could even be your own body weight). There are a few ways to represent tempo, but for our purposes we're going to use a four-number system that is a modified version of Charles Poliquin's (*German Body Comp Program*, 1994) and Everett Aabarg's work (*Muscle Mechanics, 2nd Edition*, 2006 and *Resistance Training Instruction*, 1999) on the subject. Each number represents the time in seconds that you should stay in that phase of the movement. For example, in a dumbbell flat chest press exercise using a 3-0-1-0 tempo scheme, the first *3* is the lowering of the weight down to your chest, the second *0* represents the pause at the bottom, the *1* is how quickly you push the weight back up above your chest, and the last *0* represents the hold at the top before repeating. Of course, a *0* means that you don't pause in that phase and should continue right into the next phase of the exercise. Those four numbers are also called the positive (or concentric) phase, the negative (or eccentric) phase, and the two peak positions of the concentric and eccentric phases. We're not going to get too deep into your tempo, but you should keep in mind that the weight should move quickly when you're trying to move it and then slow down when it's coming back to its starting position.

• **Rest**: Rest refers to the amount of time that you'll have between sets. So the chart entry *90 s* means after you drop the weights after your last set, you can begin resting for 90 seconds before starting the next round. It also means that there will be no more 10-minute breaks hanging around the water cooler or chatting it up with your buddies or the ladies at the front desk. You'll have plenty of time for that after the workout, but for the next 30 to 45 minutes it's game time!

USING CHARTS TO TRACK YOUR PROGRESS

I've noticed that many strength and conditioning coaches and personal trainers have gotten away from keeping a clipboard near them during their clients' workouts. I can't understand why this trend has started, because if you don't track your numbers, you won't be able to know whether you're improving.

You must either take this book with you to the gym and use the charts supplied in it or transfer the exercises into a small notebook and use that. Either way, you must track your progress.

You've seen guys in the gym who have been doing the same thing and lifting the same weights for the last five years and they're wondering why they haven't gotten the results that they're looking for. Don't be one of those guys.

I'm going to make the chart simple to use, and I think that you'll have fun filling it in. My studio and online clients enjoy checking their numbers after each workout to see how they've improved. Remember, with short four- to six-week workout plans your goal is to improve from one week to the next. When you plateau, it's time to move on to the next six-week exercise routine written up for you.

Table 4.1 on page 36 shows a sample workout chart like the ones that you'll be using. But before we get to it you'll want to understand a few items to ease the transition to using this type of chart. You'll first notice that the exercises are all written in the first column. After about two or three exercises, you will see an empty line, which indicates that the preceding block of exercises are meant to be done back to back without more than a few seconds of rest between them.

You'll also see instructions in parentheses that let you know how long you should rest before completing the preceding block of exercises again. You move on to the next grouping of exercises after you have completed the specified number of rounds or sets.

Table 4.1 Strength-Training Workout 1

Exercise	Sets	Reps	Tempo	Week 1	Week 2	Week 3	Week 4	Week 5	Week 6
Warm-up exercise 1	1	12	1-1-1	Weights					
				Body weight					
Warm-up exercise 2	1	2 x 12	1-1-1	6					
Warm-up exercise 3	1	AMAP	1-0-1	60 s					
(Once warm-up exercises are completed, begin strength training.)									
Strength exercise 1									
Strength exercise 2									
(Rest 90 s and repeat exercises 1 and 2.)									
Strength exercise 3									
Strength exercise 4									
(Rest 90 s and repeat exercises 3 and 4.)									
Strength exercise 5									
Strength exercise 6									
(Rest 90 s and repeat exercises 5 and 6.)									

Beside the exercises you'll see a column for the corresponding number of sets for each particular exercise. You'll do most warm-ups only once, but you'll perform your major exercises three to five times.

The next column tells you how many repetitions you should do for each set. The first number indicates the number of reps for the first set. The second number refers to the second set and so on. The entry *AMAP* means that you should try for "as many (reps) as possible."

The fourth column refers to your tempo and the speed at which you should move the weight during each set.

The last six columns are for you to write in your weights each week. For the first week you should start light and find the right weight for you to complete each exercise. The first week of any new program is an unloading week, so you should allow yourself to ease into the new exercises. Some exercises are done with just your own body weight. For those movements you write in just the number of reps that you completed or the time that you held the exercise.

WHEN TO TAKE TIME OFF

Taking time off is one of the big secrets to reaping the benefits of a lifetime of strength training.

Most of us have learned this the hard way, but going too hard for too long is a surefire way to get injured. Before the age of 22 I had my fair share of injuries, but I learned from all my mistakes along the way, and I can say that I've been injury free ever since.

Although injuries and accidents can occur, this book will show you how to minimize the risks associated with any strenuous weight-bearing activity. First, you'll want to use correct form, as explained throughout the book. Second, you'll want to observe the simple guide that follows to get proper rest and recovery. Besides getting adequate nutrition and sleep, which will help your body recover at a faster rate, you'll want to build a few unloading and recovery weeks into your yearly workout plans.

As mentioned earlier, during an unloading week you take your training intensity down a notch. Typically, this means lifting lighter weights or doing fewer sets or reps. For our programs, what we're going to do is simplify the process and use just the first week of any new program as an unloading week. So in this way what you're going to do is use lighter weights and focus just on form. You should not take any exercise to failure, and you may do one less set per exercise that week.

Also, every 12 weeks you should take a full week off to give your nervous system, muscles, and joints some well-deserved rest, recovery, and rejuvenation. Even if you don't want to stop for a full week, the rest is still mandatory. You don't have to sit on your couch the whole week because you can still be active and enjoy some light sporting activities outside the gym, but you should give the weights a rest.

This full week off four times per year will serve you well in the long term.

Another thing to keep in mind is that many of us have work trips or vacations that may force us to take some time off from our workouts anyway. I suggest using this time as your recovery week and then picking right back up when you get back.

GETTING IN THE ZONE

Now let's talk about getting pumped up for your workouts!

First things first—your workouts are going to be short, intense, and to the point, so there's no room for moving through them slowly or without focus. You're going to need to bring your A game to every workout, and I have a few tips to help you get there.

If one of your primary goals is to burn body fat, you're not going to want to eat for about 90 minutes before your workout, but for anyone else I suggest a protein shake with some fruit. Also, if you're feeling low that particular day, you may want to enjoy a green tea 30 minutes before hitting the gym. The moderate caffeine infusion should help to boost your energy and will even help with your fat-burning potential during the workout. Unlike most other caffeinated and acidic beverages like coffee or energy drinks, green tea has a number of beneficial health qualities stemming from its high antioxidant properties, making it the clear winner when you need a boost.

Many clients put on an MP3 player before starting their workouts and listen to some of their favorite music. That helps many guys get motivated.

For those days when you just really don't feel like working out because you're stressed, tired, or in a bad mood, I suggest using the five-minute countdown. For this approach you make a deal with yourself that if after getting changed and working out for five minutes you still don't feel like working out, you can take the day off and just try again the next day.

The reason that I've found this tactic to work well is that the hardest part of working out is getting yourself to that first set!

On the days where you're dragging, just turn off your mind, make your protein shake, and get into your workout clothes. Before you know it you're doing your first warm-up set. And from there, you're ready to get in a great workout.

Also, there's nothing like the feeling that you get when you finish a powerful exercise session. You just feel proud to have done something good for yourself that you know most people would never even attempt.

Finally, just remember that the whole workout is going to take you only about 45 minutes and that you are receiving a lifetime of benefits that will increase the quality of your life and allow you to enjoy more health and vitality because of the decision you made to become stronger and fitter.

You are the role model that others will look up to.

FIVE SIMPLE STEPS TO GETTING RESULTS

As you've probably noticed by now, I'm big on taking the seemingly complex and breaking it down to a simple, step-by-step process. I've found that the best way to cut down on feeling overwhelmed by any undertaking is to chop up the task into smaller, more manageable pieces. Beginning a new weightlifting program is no different.

So, without further ado, here are the five steps to getting results:

Step 1: Complete three days of strength training.

Step 2: Complete one or two interval cardio days.

Step 3: Restore your body through daily stretching and self-myofascial release.

Step 4: Regenerate through proper nutrition and rest.

Step 5: Track your progress and be consistent.

If you follow those five simple steps, I have no doubt that you will excel in your new strength-training and conditioning program!

THE IDEAL WORKOUT WEEK

Now that we know what is needed to maximize results, let's continue with our pattern of simplifying the complex and outline the ideal workout week.

Ideal Workout Week

Monday: *Strength-training workout 1*

Tuesday: *Interval cardio session 1*

Wednesday: *Strength-training workout 2*

Thursday: Rest (three Rs)

Friday: *Strength-training workout 3*

Saturday: *Interval cardio session 2*

Sunday: Rest (three Rs)

This seven-day week can be customized to suit your work schedule and commitments, but you should follow its general pattern. The pattern includes no more than three days of working out in a row and ideally has a day between strength workouts. Doing strength workouts on two consecutive days is OK if the alternative is skipping one for the week, but you should try to space out workout sessions appropriately for maximum results.

The interval cardio sessions are optional and are included in each program to promote greater body transformation if that is your goal. These short interval sprint-based programs allow you to burn more body fat and tone up your muscles faster than you have in the past. Remember that the interval workouts I have planned for you aren't the typical long, slow, boring cardio sessions. These interval-based sprints are built to spike your metabolism and leave you burning fat for up to 31 hours. They're also a fantastic way to improve your cardiovascular capacity and improve overall health.

If you're naturally on the thinner side (ectomorph), you should stick with an every-other-day routine to allow proper recovery between workouts. This recovery day enables your body to repair and rebuild your muscles, which is your goal. Many people make the mistake of thinking that more is better, but if you are naturally thin you need to fight the urge to work out more. Doing so will hinder you in reaching your goal of gaining muscle.

Although your chronological age can vary significantly from your biological age, if you are in your 40s or later or don't get enough sleep, you should stick with an every-other-day routine as well. The day off between workout sessions will give your body sufficient recovery time and prevent overtraining. In the long run you'll feel younger and more energetic, and your body will look better than ever!

Lastly, I should mention that each workout has a built-in dynamic warm-up. Therefore, the workouts do not require a general warm-up such as walking on a treadmill or riding an upright bike (although you are still welcome to do these things for 5 to 10 minutes if you enjoy them and think that they benefit you).

Also, I am not recommending any specific static stretches before any of your workouts unless you think that they are necessary because of a previous injury or a buildup of scar tissue in a certain area. Again, your dynamic warm-up will actively stretch out your body, deeming any other static stretching before your session unnecessary (and potentially harmful).

But I do suggest doing a 10-minute static stretch every day. The best time to do this is directly after your workout when your muscles are most pliable. (At the end of this chapter you will find my top 10 stretches and photo demonstrations for the upper and lower body about how to complete them.) Additionally, tremendous health benefits result from performing self-myofascial-release techniques using a foam roller, as well as getting regular massages. Both of these treatments help alleviate sore muscle tissue and adhesions, and aid in many other ways to promote healing and balance within your body. Basically, what massage and self-myofascial release (which is just self-massage) do is iron out the knots in your muscles. Massage also helps restore proper length to your muscles, decrease muscle soreness, increase blood circulation, improve lymphatic flow, calm the central nervous system, and promote a host of other benefits.

MAP OUT YOUR GOALS AND STICK TO THE PLAN

In my experience a man with a plan is far more likely to achieve his goals than another without one. The man with the plan has an end in sight—something tangible that he is trying to reach. Therefore, he can set benchmarks along the way as short-term goals leading up to his long-term aspirations. The man without a plan never really knows whether he is on track to achieve anything or even what track he is on.

The first thing that you can and should do is take your baseline statistics and record the following five items every six weeks to track your progress and make sure that you are moving in the right direction.

1. **Body fat percentage**: You can have a qualified personal trainer or health professional perform a body fat analysis by using body fat calipers, water tank submersion, or bioelectrical impedance. Athletic men fall in the range of 14 to 18 percent body fat. When you begin to drop below 14 percent you will find that your abdominal muscles are more visible. Also, if your body fat is currently above 22 percent, one of your primary goals should be to get it down to at least the 22 percent mark.

2. **Circumference measurements**: Using a floppy tape measure you should measure the girth of your neck, chest, arm (flexed and at rest), waist (drawn in and at rest), hips, thigh, and calf. Choose either side of your body for the limb measurements and make sure to use that side each time.

3. **Waist-to-hip ratio**: By taking your waist measurement and dividing by your hip measurement, you can find your waist-to-hip ratio, which is one of the best indicators for a healthy heart as well as many other leading health factors (diabetes, cancers, and so on). Aim for a number below 0.95.

4. **Body mass index** (**BMI)**: Although the BMI is not as important as your body fat percentage and waist-to-hip ratio, it is a good general health reading. To find your BMI, divide your weight in kilograms by your height in meters and then divide that number by your height in meters to come up with your body mass index. Alternatively, divide your weight in pounds by height in inches, divide that number by your height in inches, and multiply by 703. A healthy BMI is between 19 and 24.9. If your BMI is higher than that but your body fat is below 18 percent, you are likely in the clear. If your BMI is above 24 and your body fat percentage is above 22 percent, you will want to aim to reduce both of those numbers over the next few months.

5. **Lean body mass**: You can easily calculate this figure after you find your body fat percentage. All you have to do is take your body fat percentage (make it a decimal) and multiply it by your weight. For example, if you weigh 185 pounds (83.9 kg) and you have 27 percent body fat, you multiply .27 by 185 to get 49.95 (or multiply .27 by 83.9 to get 22.7), which is the amount of body fat that you currently have in pounds (kg). When you subtract the 49.95 pounds (22.7 kg) from your current body weight, the remaining figure is the amount of lean body mass that you have right now. In this case the number is 135.05 (61.2).

The useful thing about figuring out this formula is that now you can scientifically calculate how much muscle you're adding (and how much fat you're losing) every six weeks without guessing. Remember, if you're adding muscle and losing body fat at the same time, the scale will not reveal the whole picture of what's going on physiologically, so it's always best to check your body fat by the same method every six weeks.

Now that you know where you stand from a baseline statistics point, let's talk about how to set goals.

I suggest writing out your long-term goals on an index card that you can keep with your workout gear. That way you can glance at it and remember why you have set forth on this path in the first place every time you get ready to challenge yourself in the weight room. An old photo of yourself, an image of the ideal body that you're aiming to achieve, or a specific amount of weight that you're looking to lift can also be added to your future vision of you.

After you have that focused vision of your long-term goals of what you would like to be, feel, and achieve, you should break them down into short-term goals. Start with one-month, three-month, and six-month goals. You may even find that after six months you've achieved all your long-term goals of body transformation.

But you should never believe that you are finished after you achieve your physical goals. Although you cannot see the inner working of your body, a healthy lifestyle that includes exercise will reward you with a stronger, healthier, and more zestful appreciation for living a fully functional life for years to come.

IT'S A WRAP

Now that we've covered everything you need to begin your new workout programs, I want to congratulate you on making it this far through the book. You wouldn't believe how many people give up before they even lace up their sneakers. You have already set yourself apart from those who just think about doing things. You have entered the elite category of those who take action and do something! To be honest, I'm excited for you because I've been in your position many times, and I continue to be at that jumping-off point every time I undertake a new adventure or challenge that I must set my mind to.

Well, enough talk. Let the workouts begin!

ADDUCTOR STRETCH

How to: Sit flat on your hips with your feet pulled in. Place the soles of your feet against each other and move your knees toward the floor. Hold on to your ankles and gently use your elbows to push your inner thighs closer to the floor.

Benefits: This stretch will help open up your inner thighs.

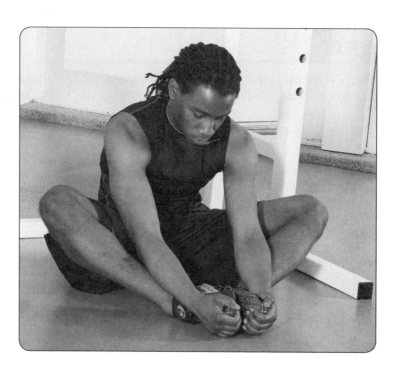

TRAINING TIP

Hold each stretch for 30 to 90 seconds. Always ease into the stretch and never bounce or hold your breath.

CROSS-LEGGED STRETCH

How to: Sit flat on your hips and cross your legs in front of you. Reach for the ceiling, bend over, and fall at the waist to the floor. Keep your hips in contact with the floor while reaching out in front of you with your arms and touching the floor.

Benefits: This stretch will open up your hips and lower back.

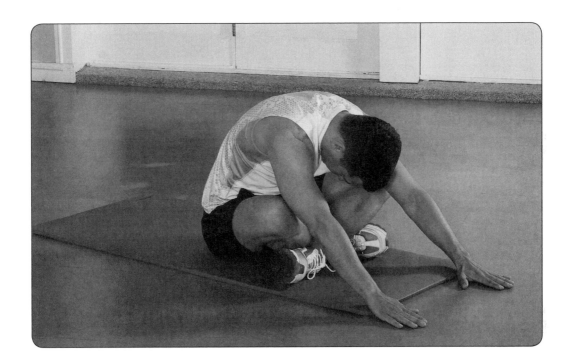

TRAINING TIP

Hold each stretch for 30 to 90 seconds. Always ease into the stretch and never bounce or hold your breath.

GLUTE STRETCH

How to: Sit flat on a mat on your hips and place your legs out straight. Slowly bend one leg up to your chest and place it over your other leg onto the floor. Make sure to keep your knee and ankle in alignment. Wrap both arms tightly around your leg and hold it into your body. Hold for 30 to 90 seconds and then repeat on the other leg.

Benefits: This stretch will help open your hip rotators and glutes.

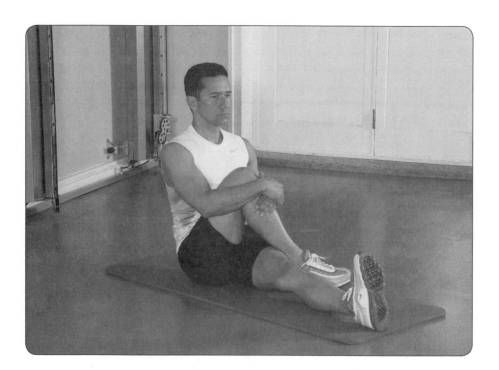

TRAINING TIP

Hold each stretch for 30 to 90 seconds. Always ease into the stretch and never bounce or hold your breath.

KNEELING LUNGE

How to: Kneel straight up on the ground on both knees. Lunge forward with one leg. Allow the front side of the kneeling leg to stretch. After you feel balanced, raise the arm on the side of the kneeling leg to enhance the stretch further. Face your palm into your head and maintain this stretch for 30 to 90 seconds. Repeat on the other side.

Benefits: This stretch will open up your hips, hip flexors, and ankles.

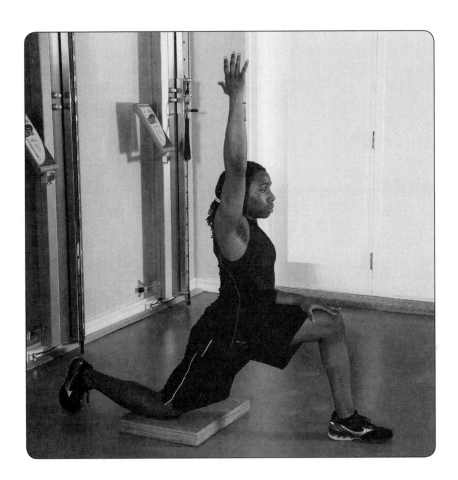

TRAINING TIP

Hold each stretch for 30 to 90 seconds. Always ease into the stretch and never bounce or hold your breath.

LYING HAMSTRING STRETCH

How to: Lie flat on your back. Place a towel or strap around the arch of your foot and slowly raise that leg up straight until you feel tension in the back of your thigh. Keep the bottom leg relatively flat on the ground. Never pull beyond where you feel tension. If the tension starts to ease, you may go deeper into the stretch. Hold for 30 to 90 seconds and then repeat on the other leg.

Benefits: This stretch will help open your hamstrings and calves.

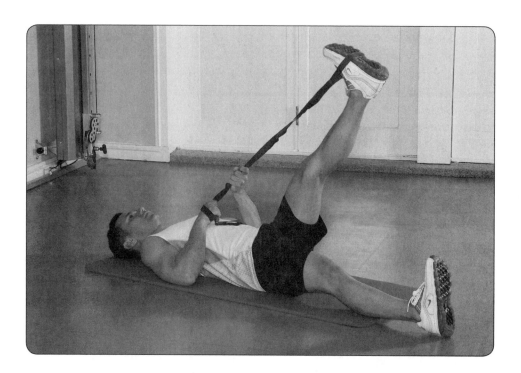

TRAINING TIP

Hold each stretch for 30 to 90 seconds. Always ease into the stretch and never bounce or hold your breath.

LYING QUADRICEPS STRETCH

How to: Lie flat on your right side with your right arm resting on the ground below your head. Reach behind you and grab your left ankle and foot as you bend your top (left) leg to your glute. Squeeze your left glute and allow your left quadriceps to stretch. Also, try to pull your heel gently away from your glute to get deeper into the stretch.

Benefits: This stretch will open up your quadriceps.

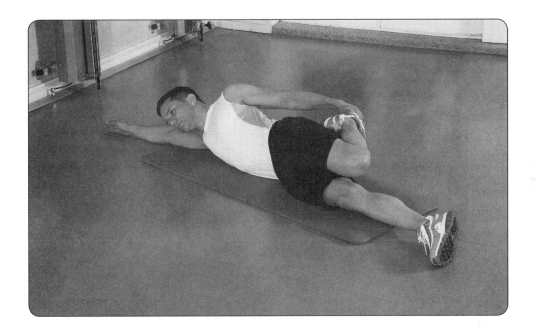

TRAINING TIP

Hold each stretch for 30 to 90 seconds. Always ease into the stretch and never bounce or hold your breath.

ONE-ARM OVERHEAD REACH

How to: Stand straight up and raise one arm overhead. Slowly lean away toward the opposite side and push your hip out. Keep your ankle, knee, hip, shoulder, and head in alignment as you reach and lean over to one side. Hold for 30 to 90 seconds and repeat on the other side.

Benefits: This stretch will elongate your lats, hips, and obliques.

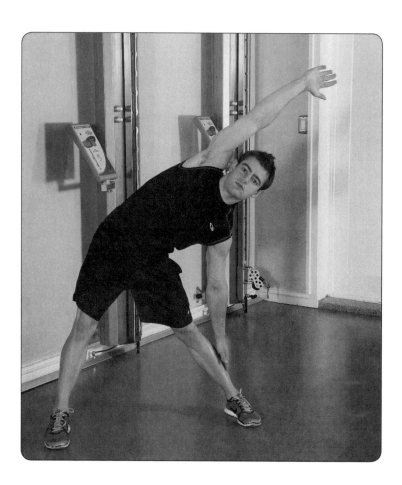

TRAINING TIP

Hold each stretch for 30 to 90 seconds. Always ease into the stretch and never bounce or hold your breath.

TRICEPS STRETCH

How to: Stand straight up and raise one arm overhead. Let that arm bend and pat yourself on the back of your shoulder. Use the other arm to help increase the stretch by easing the elbow back. Keep your head facing straight ahead and do not drop your chin into your chest. Hold for 30 to 90 seconds and repeat on the other side.

Benefits: This stretch will open up your triceps.

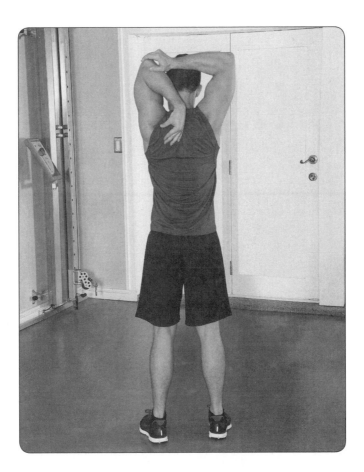

TRAINING TIP

Hold each stretch for 30 to 90 seconds. Always ease into the stretch and never bounce or hold your breath.

INTERLOCKED BICEPS STRETCH

How to: Stand up straight and fold your hands in front of you. Slowly rotate your palms away from your body. Stretch out your arms and pull downward toward the ground.

Benefits: This stretch will elongate your traps, biceps, and forearms.

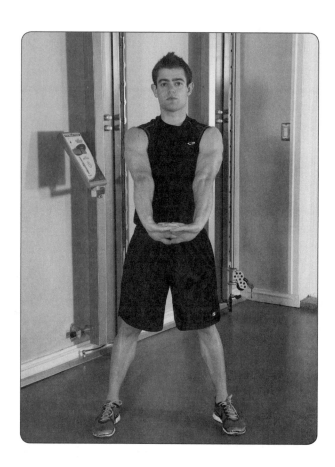

TRAINING TIP

Hold each stretch for 30 to 90 seconds. Always ease into the stretch and never bounce or hold your breath.

DOORWAY CHEST STRETCH

How to: Stand up straight and place both hands and elbows above shoulder height against a doorway frame. Slowly step through the doorway with one leg to increase the stretch. If you can't find a doorway, you may stretch one arm at a time against any sturdy object. Step out with the leg on same side as the arm that is raised.

Benefits: This stretch will open up your chest.

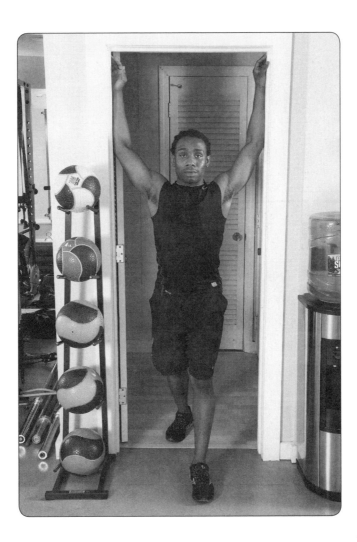

TRAINING TIP

Hold each stretch for 30 to 90 seconds. Always ease into the stretch and never bounce or hold your breath.

CHAPTER 5

Starter Program 1

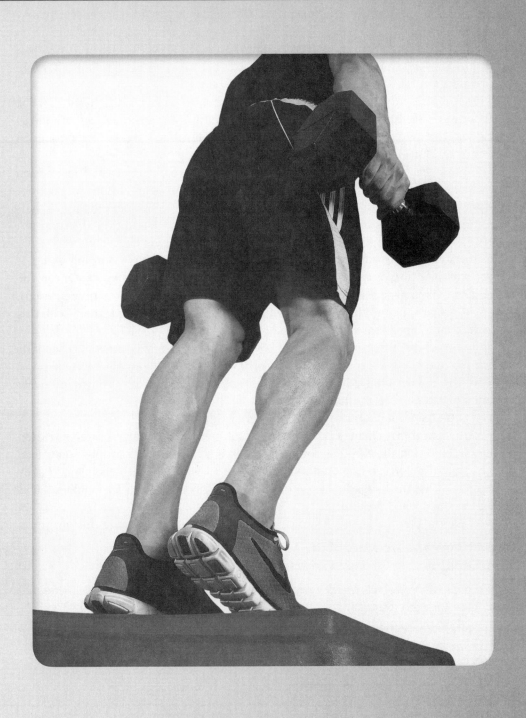

All right, it's time to get started!

This first program focuses on helping you get your body back in top shape and condition if you've taken some time off from hitting the weights at the gym. The program is also useful for anyone who is stuck at a plateau or has been doing the same group of exercises for months without any real change in exercise selection or repetition range.

I choose this foundational workout program for many of my new body transformation clients, regardless of where they're at (of course, I tweak various components based on their past injuries or current imbalances). I also like to add it in for anyone who's been doing only strength-training work because it provides a completely new stimulus.

What we're going to do in Starter Program 1 is drill down to the top functional strength-training exercises that you must master before moving on to heavier, more complex lifts.

These movements involve a full range of motion to stretch and strengthen the connective tissue surrounding your joints for maximum neuromuscular stabilization down the road when you're performing heavy dumbbell presses or one-legged movements. But I have to be upfront with you.

I do not want to give you the impression that this program is easy. I just added this same type of routine back into my personal program after about a year of not attempting these particular exercises. I've found that my shoulders, obliques, balance, and overall joint stabilization are now much stronger. In addition, the program offers another huge benefit that I haven't even touched on yet.

With each workout you're going to find that your heart rate is pumping and that you feel as if you're burning fat while working your cardiovascular system at the same time. This aspect is one of the best features of the programs that I design. You will not only be building stronger muscles but also be getting leaner. I call this type of work interval-based, metabolic resistance training.

You'll be doing three exercises in a row and spending only about 20 seconds after each one to switch movements and pick up the weights for the next exercise. So you'll be doing about 2 to 3 minutes of straight work and then resting 60 to 90 seconds to recover before the next set.

You can't help but get more ripped doing a workout like this!

For this reason my clients do little traditional, steady-state cardio, such as riding a bike, working on the elliptical, or running on a treadmill. We simply don't need it because we're boosting the metabolism for up to 31 hours with each specifically designed workout. Make sure to use table 5.1 and tables 5.2 and 5.3 on page 56 as a basis to track your workouts.

Now let's talk about the top 10 tips I want you to remember during this program.

Top 10 Tips and Benefits of the Muscular Endurance and Conditioning Starter Program 1:

1. For the first week complete one fewer set than specified (do two sets instead of three for each exercise).

2. Do not take any set to failure during the first week because we want to do an unloading week when starting a new program.

3. Use a full range of motion with each movement, but do not lose tension on the worked muscle group at any time during each rep.

4. Take the first week to find the right cable adjustments, squatting depths, and so on and then write them on your program card.

5. Focus on breathing and working on inhaling as you move with the resistance and exhaling while fighting or moving the weight (lifting).

6. Do not rest between exercises. You should take less than 20 seconds to transition from one movement to the next if you keep all your equipment for the following exercises near you.

7. Practice does not make perfect. Perfect practice makes perfect (and keeps you injury free), so focus on form with every rep.

8. Realize that you may seem out of shape during the first workout but recognize that your cardiovascular system will improve right along with your muscles. Remember, we're going to be working a different energy system than you may have been training in before, so it will need to be strengthened as well.

9. You'll see that we're doing many unilateral exercises that involve using just one side of your body at a time. We do this to train more of the core and nervous system as well as to allow your less dominant side to catch up and become stronger. The benefit is that you will have more strength and power in the long run!

10. Of course, if you ever experience any joint pain or if something doesn't feel right, you should always stop the set immediately. If you try it again with lighter resistance and still feel pain, you should discontinue that movement and see a doctor.

Table 5.1   Starter Program 1, Workout Chart 1

Exercise	Sets	Reps	Tempo	Week 1	Week 2	Week 3	Week 4	Week 5	Week 6
W1. Planks	1	12	Static	Weights					
				Body weight					
W2. Backward alternating lunges	1	20	1-1-1-1	Body weight					
W3. Squat to stands	1	10	1-2-1-2	Body weight					
(Once warm-up exercises are completed, begin strength training.)									
1A. Cable one-arm horizontal chest presses	3	12-12-12	3-0-1-1						
1B. Dumbbell Romanian deadlifts	3	12-12-12	3-0-1-1						
1C. JC band horizontal chops	3	12-12-12	1-0-1-1						
(Rest 90 s and repeat exercises 1A, 1B, and 1C.)									
2A. Cable one-arm horizontal rows	3	12-12-12	3-0-1-1						
2B. Dumbbell box front squats	3	12-12-12	3-0-1-1						
2C. Static bridging	3	60 s	1-0-1-1						
(Rest 90 s and repeat exercises 2A, 2B, and 2C.)									

Table 5.2   Starter Program 1, Workout Chart 2

Exercise	Sets	Reps	Tempo	Week 1	Week 2	Week 3	Week 4	Week 5	Week 6
W1. Plank	1	12	Static	Weights					
				Body weight					
W2. Backward alternating lunges	1	20	1-1-1-1	Body weight					
W3. Squat to stands	1	10	1-2-1-2	Body weight					
(Once warm-up exercises are completed, begin strength training.)									
1A. Dumbbell two-arm shoulder presses	3	12-12-12	3-0-1-0						
1B. Dynamic forward cone lunges	3	24-24-24	2-0-1-0						
1C. Cable lat pull-downs in a squat	3	12-12-12	3-0-1-1						
(Rest 90 s and repeat exercises 1A, 1B, and 1C.)									
2A. Dumbbell box deadlifts	3	12-12-12	3-0-1-1						
2B. Cable EZ-bar triceps press-downs	3	12-12-12	3-0-1-1						
2C. Dumbbell neutral to supinated curls	3	12-12-12	3-0-1-1						
(Rest 90 s and repeat exercises 2A, 2B, and 2C.)									

Table 5.3   Starter Program 1, Workout Chart 3

Exercise	Sets	Reps	Tempo	Week 1	Week 2	Week 3	Week 4	Week 5	Week 6
W1. Plank	1	12	Static	Weights					
				Body weight					
W2. Backward alternating lunges	1	20	1-1-1-1	Body weight					
W3. Squat to stands	1	10	1-2-1-2	Body weight					
(Once warm-up exercises are completed, begin strength training.)									
1A. Dumbbell ball chest presses	3	12-12-12	3-0-1-0						
1B. Dumbbell one-leg step-ups	3	2 x 12	2-0-1-0						
1C. Reverse crunches	3	AMAP	2-0-1-0						
(Rest 90 s and repeat exercises 1A, 1B, and 1C.)									
2A. Dumbbell one-arm bent-over rows	3	12-12-12	2-0-1-0						
2B. Dumbbell two-arm sumo deadlifts	3	12-12-12	3-0-1-1						
2C. Supermans	3	15	1-1-1-1						
(Rest 90 s and repeat exercises 2A, 2B, and 2C.)									

PLANKS

EXERCISE NOTES

The plank is the first dynamic warm-up exercise that you will complete before performing all three weight workouts in Starter Program 1.

Start

Step 1: Lie flat on a mat on your belly.

Step 2: Place your forearms and elbows below your shoulder joints.

Step 3: Draw in your core.

Midpoint

Step 4: Press your body off the floor so that only the balls of your feet, forearms, and fists are touching.

Step 5: Hold this pose isometrically for up to 60 seconds.

Finish

Step 6: Slowly lower your knees and body to the mat when finished.

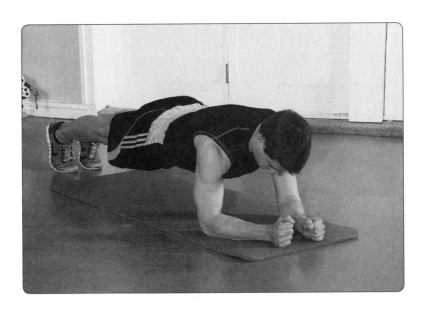

TRAINING TIP

Maintain a strong isometric position by keeping your core drawn in and your shoulders directly over your elbows.

BACKWARD ALTERNATING LUNGES

EXERCISE NOTES

- Complete the dynamic warm-up exercises first before performing all three weight workouts in Starter Program 1.
- Complete this exercise directly after performing planks.

Start

Step 1: *(a)* Stand with your feet hip-width apart and hands at your side.

Step 2: Step backward with your right leg and land on the ball of that foot.

Midpoint

Step 3: Allow your back (right) knee to bend toward the floor, stopping before it touches the ground.

Step 4: *(b)* While in your backward lunge, raise both hands overhead, stretching up straight.

Finish

Step 5: Lower your hands and step forward with your right leg so that you are back in the starting position.

Step 6: Change sides and complete the same technique with your left leg.

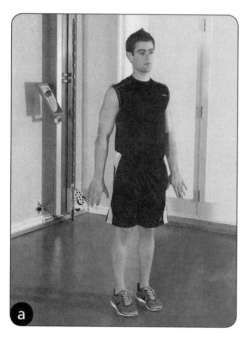
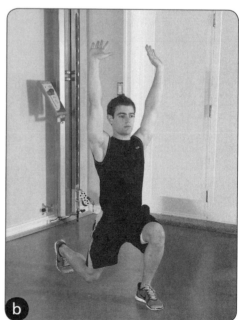

TRAINING TIP

Work on maintaining your balance and posture while trying to avoid letting your back heel touch the floor during your step back and lunge.

SQUAT TO STANDS

EXERCISE NOTES

- Complete the dynamic warm-up exercises first before performing all three weight workouts in Starter Program 1.
- Complete this exercise directly after performing backward alternating lunges.

Start

Step 1: Stand with your feet approximately hip-width apart.

Step 2: Squat down as deep as you can, keeping your heels in contact with the ground.

Step 3: *(a)* Look straight ahead, grab onto your toes, and hold them for the entire set.

Midpoint

Step 4: *(b)* Look down toward your legs and slowly straighten them, stretching your hamstrings, glutes, and lower back.

Finish

Step 5: Slowly squat back down as deep as you can, again looking straight ahead.

Step 6: Repeat and try to get slightly deeper with each stretch.

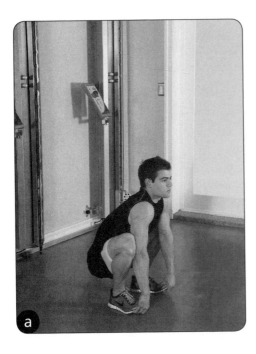 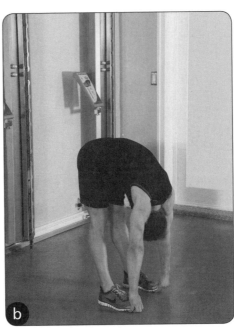

TRAINING TIP

Go as deep as you can. The goal is to be able to squat down deep enough to have your hamstrings touch your calves, as well as to straighten your legs completely on the way up.

CABLE ONE-ARM HORIZONTAL CHEST PRESSES

EXERCISE NOTES

- Complete the dynamic warm-up exercises first.
- This is the first exercise in Starter Program 1.

Start

Step 1: Grab a single cable attached at shoulder height in your left hand.

Step 2: *(a)* Step forward with your right leg into a staggered stance.

Step 3: Point your palm toward the floor and keep your wrist, elbow, and shoulder on the same plane.

Midpoint

Step 4: *(b)* Press the cable out, forcefully squeezing your left pectoral and shoulder muscles. Exhale at this point to help produce force.

Finish

Step 5: Slowly decelerate the weight back to the starting position while feeling your chest and shoulder muscles stretch.

Step 6: Repeat on the left side and then move on to the right.

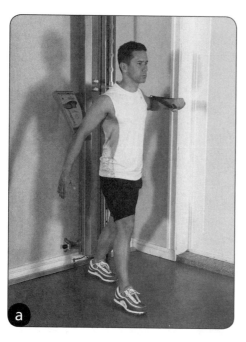 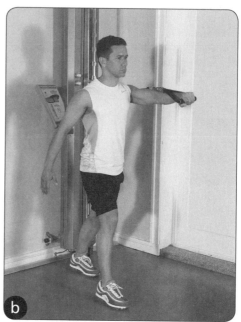

TRAINING TIP

Fight your body's inclination to twist into the cable machine as the handle is coming back into your body. Use your obliques and core to stabilize yourself and look forward.

DUMBBELL ROMANIAN DEADLIFTS

EXERCISE NOTES

- This is the second exercise in Starter Program 1.
- Complete this exercise directly after doing cable one-arm horizontal chest presses.

Start

Step 1: *(a)* Stand with your feet hip-width apart and hold a pair of dumbbells with your palms facing the sides of your body.

Step 2: Keep a slight static bend in your knees and place your body weight on your heels.

Step 3: Maintain a flat back (neutral spine) and retract your shoulder blades for posture during the entire set. Do not allow the dumbbells to swing forward during the movement (keep them beside your legs).

Midpoint

Step 4: *(b)* Allow your hips to stretch backward (without trying to bend your knees) until you can't stretch your hamstrings and glutes anymore. Your upper body will lower a little, but the hips always move first and dictate how low you go.

Finish

Step 5: Push your hips forward and pull your upper body back to the starting position before performing the next repetition. Exhale as you exert force and lift up.

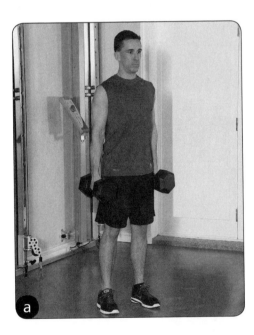 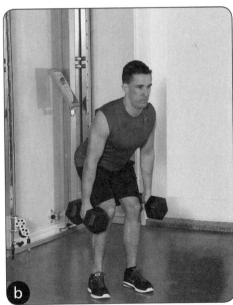

TRAINING TIP

Do not look down to the floor as you stretch back with your hips and lower the weights. This act will cause you to shift the weight off your heels and onto the balls of your feet while simultaneously rounding out your back.

JC BAND HORIZONTAL CHOPS

EXERCISE NOTES

- This is the third exercise in Starter Program 1.
- Complete this exercise directly after performing dumbbell Romanian deadlifts.
- Because this is the third exercise in your tri-set, you will rest after completing it.

Start

Step 1: Attach a JC band at shoulder height.

Step 2: Stand perpendicular to the attachment and step away from it far enough so that the band has a good amount of tension on it.

Step 3: *(a)* Clasp both handles with your hands and keep your feet shoulder-width apart.

Step 4: Keep a slight bend in your knees the entire time and engage your core.

Step 5: Keep your elbows straight but not locked out throughout the set.

Midpoint

Step 6: *(b)* Looking straight ahead and without rotating your upper body, chop your arms powerfully across your chest until the band stretches across your inside shoulder. Exhale forcefully as you chop.

Finish

Step 7: Maintain your posture and allow the band to return slowly to the starting position without twisting or losing tension.

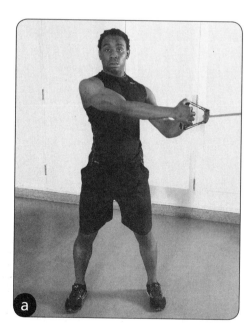 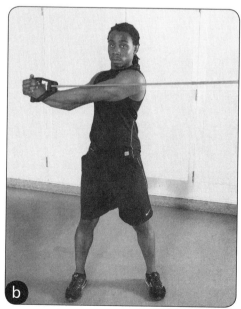

TRAINING TIP

Hold your body strong the whole time. Do not let your knees buckle in or your upper body rotate. Also, do not allow your elbows to bend excessively!

CABLE ONE-ARM HORIZONTAL ROWS

EXERCISE NOTES

- Complete the entire first tri-set two or three times before moving on to the second group of exercises.
- This is the first exercise in the second tri-set of Starter Program 1.

Start

Step 1: Grab a single cable attached at shoulder height in your left hand.

Step 2: *(a)* Step backward with your left leg into a staggered stance so that there is tension on the cable at all times.

Step 3: Point your palm toward the floor and keep your wrist, elbow, and shoulder on the same plane.

Midpoint

Step 4: *(b)* Pull the cable toward your left shoulder, forcefully squeezing the muscles on the left side of your back while stretching the muscles of your left pectorals. Exhale while pulling in.

Finish

Step 5: Slowly decelerate the weight back to the starting position while feeling your back and shoulder muscles stretch. Keep your core engaged and your legs rooted into the ground to prevent your body from being pulled forward toward the weight stack. Breathe in as the weight returns to its starting position.

Step 6: Repeat on the left side and then move on to the right.

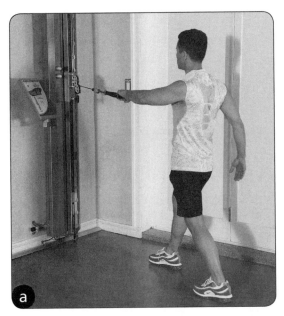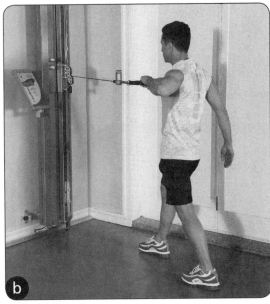

TRAINING TIP

Use your obliques, core, and legs to stabilize your entire body while looking at the cable attachment in front of you throughout the set.

DUMBBELL BOX FRONT SQUATS

EXERCISE NOTES

- This is the second exercise in the second tri-set of Starter Program 1.
- Complete this exercise directly after performing cable one-arm horizontal rows.

Start

Step 1: Grab a pair of dumbbells and hold them by your sides.

Step 2: Stand about 4 inches (10 cm) in front of a box that is about the height of your knees.

Step 3: *(a)* Place and balance both dumbbells up on your shoulders.

Midpoint

Step 4: Keeping your core engaged, sit back with your hips while maintaining good posture and keeping your chest up.

Step 5: *(b)* Slowly sit down on the box without disengaging your core.

Finish

Step 6: Drive through your heels while exhaling and push your body back to a standing position.

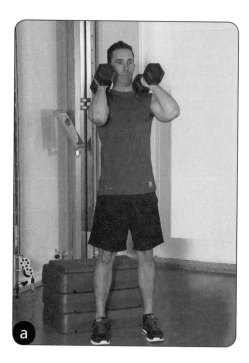 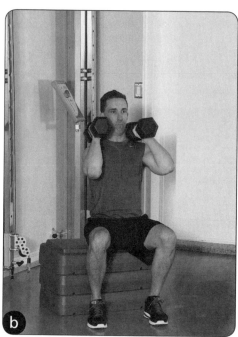

TRAINING TIP

Keep the weight back on your heels and do not allow your knees to cheat forward over your toes. Just keep pushing back with your hips, knowing that you have the box there as your safety net to practice great form.

STATIC BRIDGING

EXERCISE NOTES

- This is the third exercise in the second tri-set of Starter Program 1.
- Complete this exercise directly after performing dumbbell box front squats.
- Because this is the third exercise in your tri-set, you will rest after completing it.

Start

Step 1: Lie on your back.

Step 2: Pull both feet into your hips.

Step 3: Keep your arms flat on the floor (beginner), or place your hands on your chest but keep your elbows on the floor (intermediate), or fold your arms across your chest (advanced).

Step 4: Keep your knees directly over your ankles and your feet flat on the floor.

Step 5: Engage your glutes by squeezing them together.

Midpoint

Step 6: Keeping your glutes engaged throughout the set, lift your hips off the floor.

Finish

Step 7: Maintain a straight line from your shoulders to your knees.

Step 8: Breathe naturally and hold this position for up to 60 seconds.

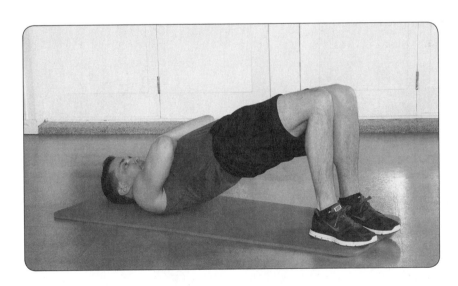

TRAINING TIP

Hold a towel or small ball between your knees to disable your body's inclination to allow your knees to flare out. Also, if your hamstrings cramp up or you begin to feel it too much in that area or your lower back, remember to keep squeezing the glutes together to make them the dominant hip extensor.

DUMBBELL TWO-ARM SHOULDER PRESSES

EXERCISE NOTES

- Complete the dynamic warm-up exercises first.
- This is the first exercise in the second workout of Starter Program 1.

Start

Step 1: Stand with your feet shoulder-width apart holding a pair of dumbbells by your sides.

Step 2: Keep your knees bent and your core engaged throughout the set.

Step 3: *(a)* Lift both dumbbells about 2 inches (5 cm) above your shoulders and face your palms away from your body.

Midpoint

Step 4: *(b)* Press the dumbbells directly overhead without rotating your wrists or arching your back.

Finish

Step 5: Slowly decelerate the weight back to the starting position above your shoulders while keeping tension on the deltoids.

Step 6: Maintain form and repeat.

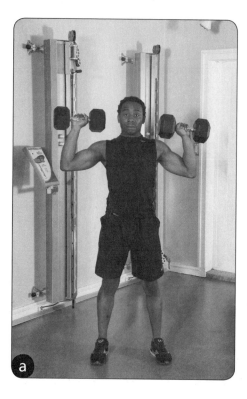
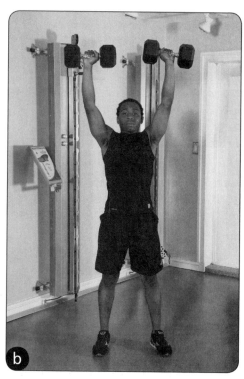

TRAINING TIP

Fight your body's inclination to arch backward and turn the exercise into a modified chest press. Engage your abs and core and maintain proper posture.

DYNAMIC FORWARD CONE LUNGES

EXERCISE NOTES

- This is the second exercise in the second workout of Starter Program 1.
- Complete this exercise directly after performing dumbbell two-arm shoulder presses.

Start

Step 1: *(a)* Stand with your feet hip-width apart with your arms raised overhead and position yourself about half your body's length away from a 12-inch (30 cm) cone or object in front of you.

Step 2: Step forward with your left leg while keeping the weight on the front heel and sitting onto the front left hip.

Midpoint

Step 3: Allow your right knee to bend straight down to the ground and stop 3 to 4 inches (8 to 10 cm) before touching the floor.

Step 4: *(b)* Without excessively dropping your upper body forward, lower your arms to touch the top of the cone with both hands.

Finish

Step 5: Push through your left heel while raising your arms overhead back to the original starting position.

Step 6: Alternate sides with each repetition.

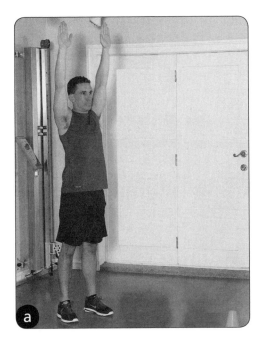
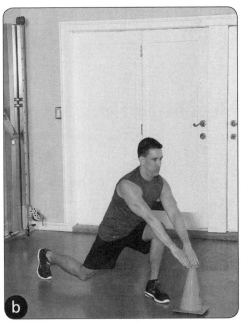

TRAINING TIP

Do not allow your weight to shift onto the ball of the front foot or let your front knee go over your toes. You should sit into the lunge by placing the weight on your front hip and heel.

CABLE LAT PULL-DOWNS IN A SQUAT

EXERCISE NOTES

- This is the third exercise in the second workout of Starter Program 1.
- Complete this exercise directly after performing dynamic forward cone lunges.
- Because this is the third exercise in your tri-set, you will rest after completing it.

Start

Step 1: Attach two handles to two high-cable pulleys slightly wider than shoulder-width apart. Even wider is fine, but closer than shoulder-width apart will not work.

Step 2: *(a)* Grab both handles with outstretched arms and sit back into a half squat.

Step 3: Keep both palms facing directly away from you throughout the set as you begin to pull the handles down forcefully to the sides of your shoulders. Aim to touch your thumbs to the sides of your shoulders.

Midpoint

Step 4: *(b)* Maintain your squat and look straight ahead as you squeeze your lats (the muscles under your armpits), holding the handles to your shoulders.

Finish

Step 5: Begin to allow the weights to return slowly to the starting position while holding your squat position.

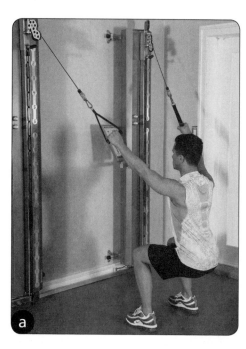
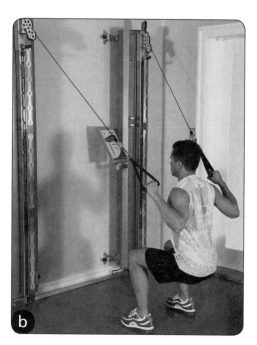

TRAINING TIP

Do not make the mistake of turning this exercise into a biceps movement in which you neglect your back muscles and simply muscle the weight down by flexing your biceps. You can easily avoid this by not allowing your palms to turn into your body or by not pulling the handles to your chest. Instead, retract your shoulder blades and pull them down and back.

DUMBBELL BOX DEADLIFTS

EXERCISE NOTES

- Complete the entire first tri-set of the second workout two or three times before moving on to the second group of exercises.
- This is the first exercise in the second tri-set of the second workout.

Start

Step 1: *(a)* Grab a pair of dumbbells and hold them by your sides.

Step 2: Stand about 4 inches (10 cm) in front of a box that is about the height of your knees.

Step 3: Lift your chest up and retract your shoulder blades.

Midpoint

Step 4: Keeping your core engaged, sit back with your hips while maintaining good posture and keeping your weight on your heels.

Step 5: *(b)* Slowly sit down on the box without disengaging your core.

Finish

Step 6: Drive through your heels while exhaling and push your body back to a standing position.

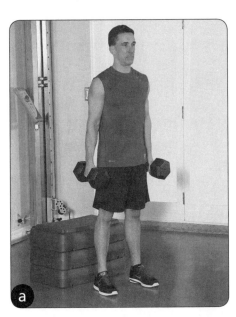 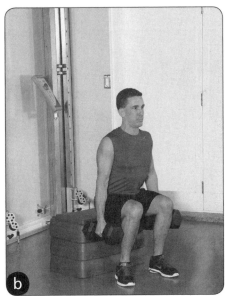

TRAINING TIP

If my clients aren't used to going that deep, I really like having them use the knee-height box to work on squatting to parallel while performing this deadlift because there is a safety net to catch them. The exercise stretches and activates more muscle fiber and gives you far better results. Just make sure that you sit back on your hips and heels and don't let your knees go over your toes. This rule goes for every leg exercise.

Side note: Many people refer to this exercise as a dumbbell squat, but if you were to replace the dumbbells with a barbell you would be completing an Olympic deadlift. Just using dumbbells doesn't make it a squat; you're still pulling the weight from the floor.

CABLE EZ-BAR TRICEPS PRESS-DOWNS

EXERCISE NOTES

- This is the second exercise of the second tri-set of the second workout.
- Complete this exercise directly after performing dumbbell box deadlifts.

Start

Step 1: Attach an EZ-bar to a cable above your head height.

Step 2: Stand in a staggered stance with your knees bent.

Step 3: *(a)* Use an overhand close grip, and pull the bar to your chest.

Midpoint

Step 4: *(b)* Keeping your core engaged and your elbows in line with your wrists and shoulders, squeeze the weight straight down in front of you until you complete a controlled lock out of your triceps.

Step 5: Squeeze your triceps at the bottom of the movement without leaning your chest forward.

Finish

Step 6: Slowly allow the weight to return to the starting position by letting your forearms touch your biceps and without allowing your elbows to come away from your body.

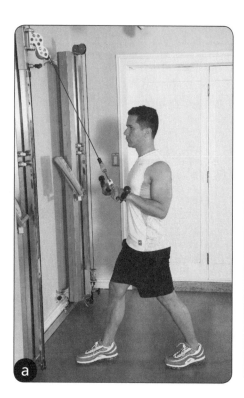
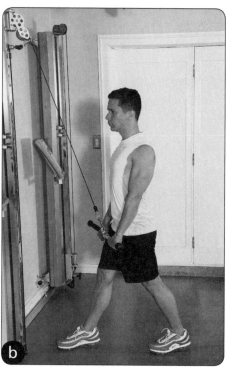

TRAINING TIP

Don't sacrifice form for loading up a lot of weight on the cable machine. This approach will lead only to elbow injuries, poor form, and less muscle development.

DUMBBELL NEUTRAL TO SUPINATED CURLS

EXERCISE NOTES

- This is the third exercise in the second tri-set of the second workout.
- Complete this exercise directly after performing cable EZ-bar triceps press-downs.
- Because this is the third exercise in your tri-set, you will rest after completing it.

Start

Step 1: *(a)* Stand with your feet hip-width apart holding a pair of dumbbells facing your sides (neutral grip means that the palms are facing each other; also referred to as a parallel grip).

Step 2: Keep your chest up, shoulder blades retracted, knees bent, and chin parallel to the ground throughout the set.

Step 3: Moving just your forearms, rotate both dumbbells as you curl so that your palms face up. Exhale at this point to help produce more force.

Midpoint

Step 4: *(b)* Squeeze your biceps forcefully without allowing your elbows to pull forward or your shoulder blades to round.

Finish

Step 5: Slowly allow the weight to return to the starting position by letting your forearms rotate back to a neutral grip by your sides.

Step 6: Before your biceps and forearms lose tension begin your next repetition.

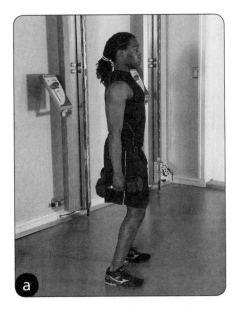
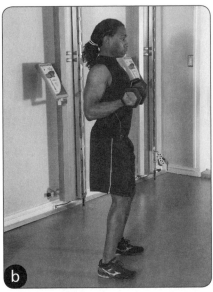

TRAINING TIP

I see many people who do not keep their hands in alignment with their forearms because they allow their wrists to "break" or bend during the curl and lowering of the weight. To keep your wrists and forearms safe and strong, make sure to maintain alignment.

DUMBBELL BALL CHEST PRESSES

EXERCISE NOTES

- Complete the dynamic warm-up exercises first.
- This is the first exercise in the third workout of Starter Program 1.

Start

Step 1: Sit on a stability ball and hold a pair of dumbbells on your quadriceps.

Step 2: Bring the dumbbells into your chest as you begin to walk your feet out in front of you and roll out on the ball.

Step 3: Stop when the ball is touching only the back of your head and upper back. Make sure to engage your core and squeeze your glutes together to form a strong bridge that you can maintain throughout the set.

Step 4: *(a)* Turn your palms out to face away from you and hold the dumbbells about 1 to 2 inches (2.5 to 5 cm) over the front of your shoulders.

Midpoint

Step 5: *(b)* Exhale, press the dumbbells up in an arc directly over your shoulders, and squeeze your chest muscles together, bringing the weights closer to each other.

Finish

Step 6: Slowly decelerate the weight back to the starting position above your shoulders while stretching and keeping tension on your chest.

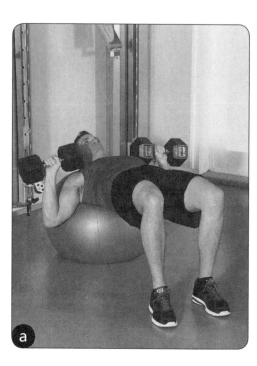 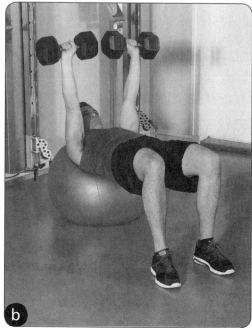

TRAINING TIP

Make sure not to rest your arms on the ball on the way down. Keep tension on your chest throughout the set!

DUMBBELL ONE-LEG STEP-UPS

EXERCISE NOTES

- This is the second exercise in the third workout of Starter Program 1.
- Complete this exercise directly after performing dumbbell ball chest presses.

Start

Step 1: Place a box or bench that is approximately knee height on the floor in front of you.

Step 2: Hold a pair of dumbbells by your sides with your shoulders pulled back and your chest lifted.

Step 3: *(a)* Place your left foot up on the box and leave your right foot on the ground.

Midpoint

Step 4: *(b)* Keep the weight on your left heel and push up through the foot and hip until you are standing up straight on top of the box.

Finish

Step 5: Slowly decelerate your right leg back down to the floor without taking the tension off your left hip. Do not rock backward when you land; keep the weight on the front (left) leg, which is up on the box.

Step 6: Repeat for the desired number of repetitions and then switch legs and begin stepping up with the right leg.

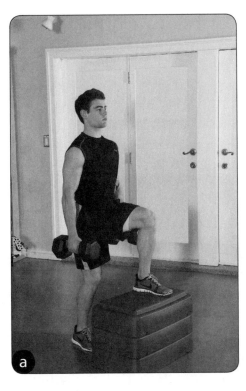 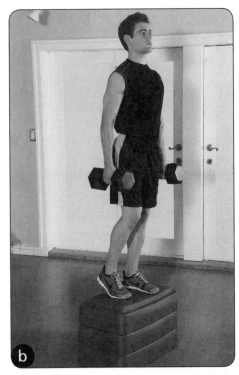

TRAINING TIP

For the best results just tap the trailing leg on top of the box with the ball of that foot as you reach the top. When you step back down with that trailing leg, make sure not to shift all the weight onto it and lose the tension on the front leg.

REVERSE CRUNCHES

EXERCISE NOTES

- This is the third exercise in the third workout of Starter Program 1.
- Complete this exercise directly after performing the dumbbell one-leg step-ups.
- Because this is the third exercise in your tri-set, you will rest after completing it.

Start

Step 1: Lie flat on your back with your legs outstretched (you can use a thin mat if you'd like).

Step 2: Place both hands directly under your hips to support your lower back.

Step 3: *(a)* Lift both legs 6 inches (15 cm) off the floor.

Midpoint

Step 4: *(b)* Use your entire core and focus on contracting your abs and drawing your knees above your belly.

Finish

Step 5: Slowly extend your legs back to the starting position while keeping your core engaged; do not arch your back.

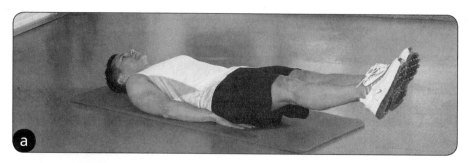

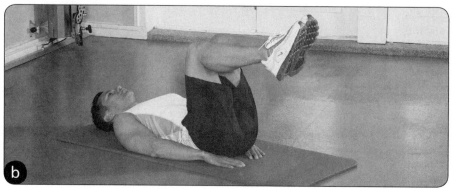

TRAINING TIP

If you find this exercise too challenging, do not extend your legs fully; keep them bent the entire time and use a shorter range of motion. If you find the exercise too easy, you may do the advanced version, called bench leg lifts. Bench leg lifts (as shown on page 100) are a similar exercise, but in this movement you slowly lower your straightened legs from above your hips to just above the floor.

DUMBBELL ONE-ARM BENT-OVER ROWS

EXERCISE NOTES

- Complete the entire first tri-set of the third workout two or three times before moving on to the second group of exercises.
- This is the first exercise in the second tri-set of the third workout.

Start

Step 1: Grab a single dumbbell in your left hand and let it hang by your side.

Step 2: Place your right hand on a sturdy weight bench or support that is at knee height.

Step 3: *(a)* Walk your right foot into the weight bench and your place your left foot behind you in a staggered stance.

Step 4: With a flat back and retracted shoulder blades, lean forward at a 45-degree angle.

Step 5: Allow the weight in your left hand to hang straight down but keep your left shoulder blade retracted so that you are not being pulled down; control the weight.

Midpoint

Step 6: *(b)* Row the weight up toward your oblique by using the muscles on the left side of your back. Do not twist your body or curl the weight up toward your chest using your biceps.

Finish

Step 7: Keep a tight grip and control the weight back down to the starting position without rounding your back.

Step 8: Repeat for the desired number of reps and switch sides.

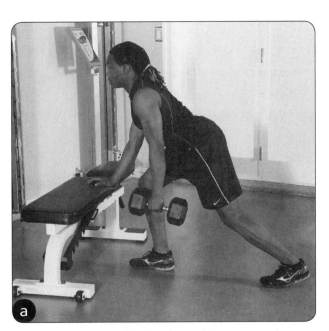

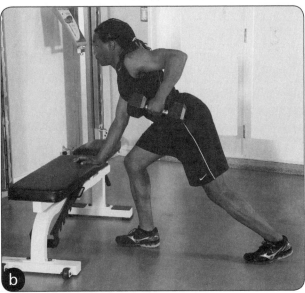

TRAINING TIP

I prefer to have my clients grab a dumbbell rack with one hand and have both feet placed firmly on the floor. This stance allows them to engage their core to a greater degree (especially the obliques) and promotes a more realistic and functional movement.

DUMBBELL TWO-ARM SUMO DEADLIFTS

EXERCISE NOTES

- This is the second exercise in the third workout of Starter Program 1.
- Complete this exercise directly after performing dumbbell one-arm bent-over rows.

Start

Step 1: *(a)* Grab a pair of dumbbells and allow them to rest against the top of your quadriceps. Your arms should remain straight for the entire set.

Step 2: Open your legs and stand in a sumo stance with your feet wider than shoulder-width apart.

Step 3: Grip the weights tightly, keep your shoulder blades pulled back, and do not round your back at any point during the movement.

Midpoint

Step 4: *(b)* Sitting back with your hips, keep your chest up and the weight on your heels. Squat down as deep as you can without letting your knees go over your toes or your back to round. Allow the dumbbells to hang between your legs as you squat down.

Finish

Step 5: Drive through your heels and glutes and push yourself while pulling the weights back up to the starting position.

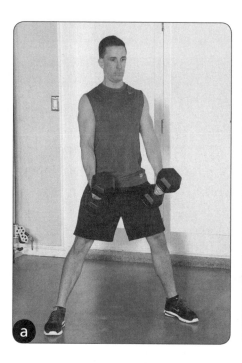 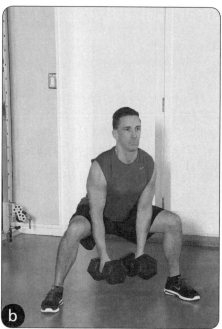

TRAINING TIP

I know it's just semantics, but this is a deadlift, not a squat, because you are pulling from the ground up (go back to the barbell analogy). Also, the best thing that you can do to keep your lower back safe during a deadlift is to keep your chest up, your shoulder blades retracted, the weight back on your heels, and your eyes looking straight ahead the whole time.

SUPERMANS

EXERCISE NOTES

- This is the third exercise in the second tri-set of the third workout.
- Complete this exercise directly after performing dumbbell two-arm sumo deadlifts.
- Because this is the third exercise in your tri-set, you will rest after completing it.

Start

Step 1: Lie flat on your belly on the floor (you can use a thin cushioned mat if you'd prefer).

Step 2: Stretch out both your arms and your legs.

Step 3: Looking straight down at the ground, lift both arms and legs off the ground 1 inch (2.5 cm) to begin to place tension on your posterior chain (the muscles on your backside).

Midpoint

Step 4: Squeeze your glutes to lift your legs (including your quads) as far off the ground as you can while squeezing your upper back at the same time to lift your chest and arms. Do not pull your head up; keep looking at the floor below you.

Finish

Step 5: Still keeping your arms and legs straight and fully extended, begin to lower your limbs in a controlled manner to the starting position 1 inch (2.5 cm) above the floor.

Step 6: Repeat.

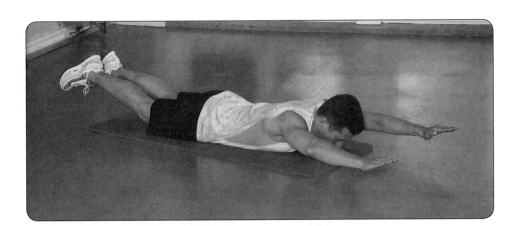

TRAINING TIP

I see many people move super fast through this exercise by using momentum instead of muscle to complete each rep. Don't be that guy—it will only hurt your back in the long run and it will not help to strengthen weak posterior chain muscles. Complete each rep deliberately and slowly to get the most out of each set. You may be able to do only a few reps until you become stronger.

CHAPTER 6

Starter Program 2

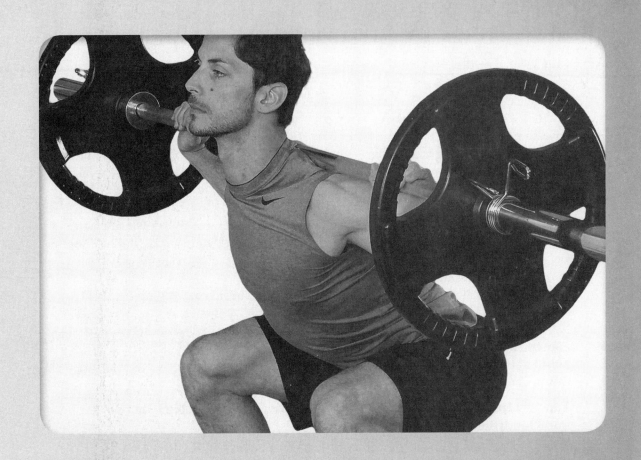

Your second starter program picks right up where the first one left off, and it offers a complete set of movements complementary to Starter Program 1. Multiple planes of movement will be introduced in this next six weeks, a period during which you can easily achieve additional strength gains. The exercise difficulty will increase, and greater neurological adaptations will force you to improve your athletic ability and range of motion.

An additional benefit of this athletic strength program will be hypertrophy. The new exercise movements will cause new growth in both the myofibrils and sarcoplasm of the muscles through increased workload and neurological recruitment. For our purposes, the myofibrils represent the muscle tissue growth itself, whereas the sarcoplasm refers to the increased swelling of the intercellular fluid in your muscle cells. I will help you achieve this through carefully designed tri-sets meant to boost your metabolic rate while improving every aspect of your athletic ability. The result will be a leaner, stronger, and better-conditioned body than you own right now!

Although my goal is to help you train like an athlete to improve your game, you don't have to be competing in any sport right now. Maybe you just play some pick-up basketball or like to toss around the football on the weekends. Whatever your level of athleticism, this program will make you more well rounded. Make no mistake about it—after training with this program for four to six weeks you'll feel like real athlete, whether you are or not!

One of the best things about strength training is that you don't necessarily have to be preparing for an event or competition. All you have to do is compete against yourself in the weight room, and your results will astound you. If you hit 55-pound (25 kg) dumbbells last week, shoot for 60 this week. Each new week of your program provides you an opportunity to excel and be your best for those 45 minutes in the gym. Stay focused on that week's goal to better yourself and train hard. With a mind-set like that, you'll notice serious body transformation results when you look in the mirror and powerful strength gains when you hit the weights. Make sure to use table 6.1 and tables 6.2 and 6.3 on page 82 as a basis to track your workouts.

Of course, at the same time I want you to keep in mind that you're in this for the long run and you have to make smart decisions when attempting new lifts. Never be afraid to push yourself, but stick to gradual improvements in strength. Play by the rules, and you'll enjoy a lifetime of athletic strength and conditioning benefits! Now let's talk about the top 10 tips that I want you to remember during this program.

Top 10 Tips and Benefits of the Athletic Strength, Muscle Growth, and Conditioning Starter Program 2:

1. It's time to take all the movements from Starter Program 1 to the next level!

2. Advanced movements challenge your nervous system and increase lean body mass.

3. We'll be using tri-sets to keep your heart rate pumping and continue to improve your cardiovascular conditioning.

4. The three-set circuits are set up to function as metabolic training units that will help elevate your metabolism for hours after you finish your workout.

5. By completing this entire workout in the allotted 45-minute time span, you will be taking advantage of the escalating-density training principle of doing more work in less time, which means greater results!

6. Remember not to rest between exercises in the tri-sets (if you can) so that you continue to challenge your body and improve your cardiovascular system at the same time that you expand your strength and power.

7. Because the exercise difficulty will be increasing, you should never go too heavy or too fast with these exercises. Use the first week of the program to go light and master the techniques involved.

8. This program is designed to be done as two balanced tri-sets, so if you do not have 45 minutes that day do just two sets of each three-exercise circuit instead of three sets. Don't do just the first tri-set and skip the second.

9. Keep in mind that you may not particularly enjoy a few exercises in each program. These are the ones that you need to focus on because they typically signal weak areas that you need to develop. The bottom line is that you shouldn't skip the hard ones!

10. Because this program includes slightly greater repetitions, if you plateau in weight after four or five weeks you can move on to the next program without having to complete the six full weeks.

Table 6.1   Starter Program 2, Workout Chart 1

Exercise	Sets	Reps	Tempo	Week 1	Week 2	Week 3	Week 4	Week 5	Week 6
W1. Mountain climbers	1	30–60 s	1-1-1-1	Weights					
				Body weight					
W2. Lateral lunges	1	2 × 12	2-1-1-1						
W3. Dumbbell one-arm empty cans	1	2 × 12	2-1-1-1						
(Once warm-up exercises are completed, begin strength training.)									
1A. Cable two-arm horizontal chest presses	3	12-12-12	3-0-1-1						
1B. Barbell back squats	3	12-10	3-0-1-1						
1C. Cable low to high chops	3	12-12-12	1-0-1-0						
(Rest 90 s and repeat exercises 1A, 1B, and 1C.)									
2A. Cable two-arm horizontal rows	3	12-12-12	3-0-1-1						
2B. Dumbbell walking lunges	3	20-16	2-0-1-1						
2C. Dynamic bridging	3	15-12	2-0-1-1						
(Rest 90 s and repeat exercises 2A, 2B, and 2C.)									

Table 6.2 Starter Program 2, Workout Chart 2

Exercise	Sets	Reps	Tempo	Week 1	Week 2	Week 3	Week 4	Week 5	Week 6
W1. Mountain climbers	1	30–60 s	1-1-1-1	Weights					
				Body weight					
W2. Lateral lunges	1	2 × 12	2-1-1-1						
W3. Dumbbell one-arm empty cans	1	2 × 12	2-1-1-1						
(Once warm-up exercises are completed, begin strength training.)									
1A. Dumbbell squat presses	3	12-12-12	2-0-1-1						
1B. Chin-ups	3	AMAP	2-0-1-1						
1C. Dumbbell axe chops	3	2 × 15	1-0-1-0						
(Rest 90 s and repeat exercises 1A, 1B, and 1C.)									
2A. Dumbbell one-leg Romanian deadlifts	3		3-0-1-1						
2B. Dips	3		2-0-1-1						
2C. Dumbbell Zottman curls	3		2-0-1-1						
(Rest 90 s and repeat exercises 2A, 2B, and 2C.)									

Table 6.3 Starter Program 2, Workout Chart 3

Exercise	Sets	Reps	Tempo	Week 1	Week 2	Week 3	Week 4	Week 5	Week 6
W1. Mountain climbers	1	30–60 s	1-1-1-1	Weights					
				Body weight					
W2. Lateral lunges	1	2 × 12	2-1-1-1						
W3. Dumbbell one-arm empty cans	1	2 × 12	2-1-1-1						
(Once warm-up exercises are completed, begin strength training.)									
1A. Declined push-ups	3	AMAP	2-0-1-1						
1B. Dumbbell shoulder-loaded step-ups	3	24-24-24	2-0-1-1						
1C. Bench leg lifts	3	AMAP	2-0-1-0						
(Rest 90s and repeat exercises 1A, 1B, and 1C.)									
2A. Dumbbell two-arm bent-over rows	3	12-12-12	2-0-1-1						
2B. Dumbbell overhead squats	3	12-10	2-0-1-1						
2C. Medicine ball side-to-side rotations	3	30	1-0-1-0						
(Rest 90s and repeat exercises 2A, 2B, and 2C.)									

MOUNTAIN CLIMBERS

EXERCISE NOTES

Complete the dynamic warm-up exercises before doing all three weight workouts in Starter Program 2.

Start

Step 1: Place both hands below your shoulders as you get into push-up position on the floor.

Step 2: Align the balls of your feet under your ankles so that only your feet and hands are in contact with the ground.

Step 3: Tighten your core.

Midpoint

Step 4: *(a)* Pull one leg off the floor and draw it into your belly while the other leg remains anchored on the ground.

Step 5: *(b)* Quickly place the leg in the air back on the floor and pull the other leg off the floor and into your belly.

Finish

Step 6: Repeat this motion by rapidly bringing one leg in while the other one works to balance you along with your upper body. Move as quickly as you can for 30 to 60 seconds.

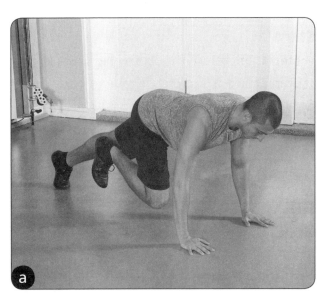
a

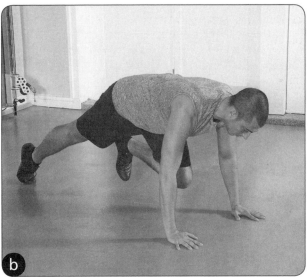
b

TRAINING TIP

To stay balanced on only three points, remember to keep your core engaged. Also, to reduce stress on your knee joint, do not allow the front foot to touch the floor when you pull it into your belly.

LATERAL LUNGES

EXERCISE NOTES

- Complete the dynamic warm-up exercises first before performing all three weight workouts in Starter Program 2.
- Complete this exercise directly after performing mountain climbers.

Start

Step 1: *(a)* Stand with your feet hip-width apart and fists raised to shoulder-height.

Step 2: Take a giant step to your right side so that your feet are parallel to each other.

Midpoint

Step 3: Absorb the landing of your right foot by keeping the weight back into your heel and decelerating into your right hip.

Step 4: *(b)* Do not allow your right knee to go over the toes of your right foot; keep sitting back into your hips. Also, straighten your left leg fully and feel the stretch on the inner thigh of that leg.

Finish

Step 5: Push through your right hip and heel and accelerate back to the starting position, bringing both feet together and standing up straight.

Step 6: Repeat on one side for the required number of repetitions and then follow the same technique on the opposite side.

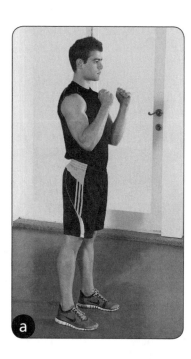
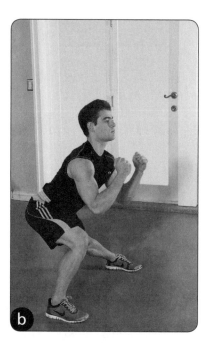

TRAINING TIP

The hardest part of this exercise is to sit back into your hips and activate your glutes. To achieve this, sit back on the heel of the foot that is lunging while making sure that the same knee does not go over your toes.

DUMBBELL ONE-ARM EMPTY CANS

EXERCISE NOTES

- Complete the dynamic warm-up exercises first before performing all three weight workouts in Starter Program 2.
- Complete this exercise directly after performing lateral lunges.

Start

Step 1: Stand with your feet shoulder-width apart and hold a dumbbell in your left hand.

Step 2: *(a)* Hold the dumbbell in front of your right hip and turn the head of the dumbbell down toward the floor by rotating your thumb to point down.

Step 3: Keep your left elbow straight but not locked throughout the set.

Midpoint

Step 4: *(b)* Raise the dumbbell up at a diagonal across your chest to about a 45-degree angle above your left shoulder. Do this by rotating your thumb so that it points directly up to the sky.

Finish

Step 5: Slowly decelerate and rotate the weight down to the starting position in front of your right hip. Your thumb and the weight will now be pointed down to the floor again.

Step 6: Repeat on the same side for the desired number of repetitions and then switch sides.

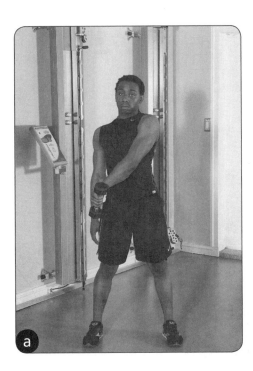 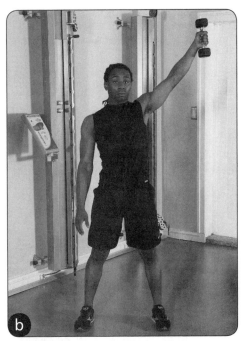

TRAINING TIP

This exercise is called an empty can because you are pretending to pour out the liquid of a can at the bottom of each rep. This exercise strengthens the muscles of the rotator cuff and gets them warmed up for your workout.

CABLE TWO-ARM HORIZONTAL CHEST PRESSES

EXERCISE NOTES

- Complete the dynamic warm-up exercises first.
- This is the first exercise in Starter Program 2.

Start

Step 1: Grab two cable handles attached at shoulder height.

Step 2: *(a)* Step forward with either leg into a staggered stance and remain there throughout the set.

Step 3: Point your palms toward the floor and keep your wrist, elbow, and shoulder on the same plane.

Midpoint

Step 4: *(b)* Press the cables out, forcefully squeezing your pectorals and the handles together. Exhale at this point to help produce force.

Finish

Step 5: Slowly decelerate the weight back to the starting position while feeling your chest and shoulder muscles stretch. Keep the tension on your chest the entire time and maintain a strong, balanced stance.

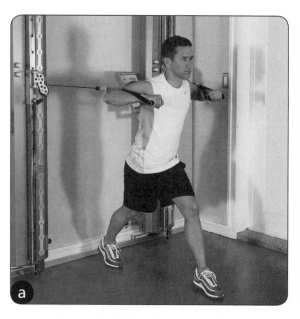 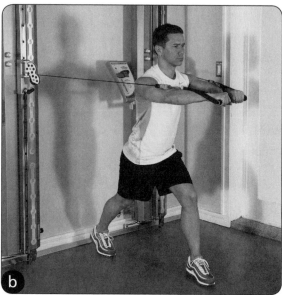

TRAINING TIP

By using both arms you will be able to decrease instability in your core and thus push more weight. Make sure to position your body as upright as possible and remember not to overextend your shoulders while pressing at chest height.

BARBELL BACK SQUATS

EXERCISE NOTES

- This is the second exercise in Starter Program 2.
- Complete this exercise directly after performing cable two-arm horizontal chest presses.

Start

Step 1: Stand with your feet shoulder-width apart and your knees slightly bent.

Step 2: *(a)* Step under the barbell and place it directly on your trapezius muscles below your neck. Hold the bar just outside shoulder-width apart.

Step 3: Maintain a flat back (neutral spine) and retract your shoulder blades for posture throughout the set. Also, make sure to keep your chest up and your chin parallel to the floor.

Midpoint

Step 4: *(b)* Slowly breathe in and sit back with your hips, keeping the weight on your heels. Get as deep as you can without rounding out your lower back, letting your heels come up, dropping your chest, or going into a posterior pelvic tilt.

Finish

Step 5: Push as hard you can through your hips and heels, propelling yourself back to the standing start position.

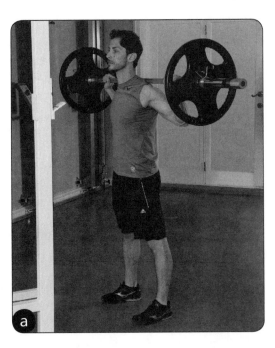
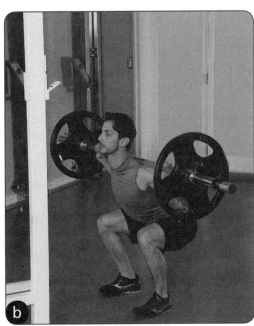

TRAINING TIP

The barbell back squat is the granddaddy of all leg exercises. You should focus on technique by starting out with lighter weight and going deeper. You'll recruit more muscle fiber this way, and as a result your legs will grow stronger more quickly. By getting to at least parallel you'll also create a far greater metabolic effect in your body.

CABLE LOW TO HIGH CHOPS

EXERCISE NOTES

- This is the third exercise in Starter Program 2.
- Complete this exercise directly after performing barbell back squats.
- Because this is the third exercise in your tri-set, you will rest after completing it.

Start

Step 1: Attach a cable handle at ankle height.

Step 2: Stand with your feet shoulder-width apart and perpendicular to the attachment (about 2 feet [60 cm] away), making sure that the cable has a good amount of tension on it.

Step 3: *(a)* Clasp the handle with both hands and interlock your fingers if possible.

Step 4: Keep a slight bend in your knees the entire time and engage your core.

Step 5: Keep your elbows straight but not locked throughout the set.

Step 6: Begin with the weight to the side of your inside leg (closer to the cable tower).

Midpoint

Step 7: *(b)* Looking straight ahead and without rotating your upper body, chop your arms powerfully up and over your outside shoulder until the cable stretches across your chest. Exhale forcefully as you chop.

Finish

Step 8: Maintain your posture and allow your arms to return slowly to the starting position without twisting your torso or losing tension.

Step 9: Repeat for the desired number of repetitions and then switch sides.

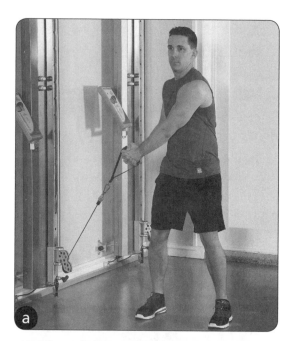

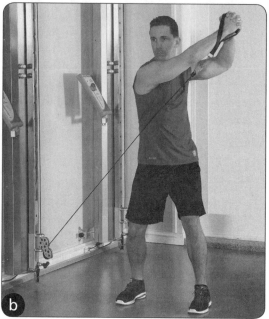

TRAINING TIP

Stand in an athletic stance and keep your knees slightly bent the entire time. Also, use the ground for power by pushing into it as you chop from low to high.

CABLE TWO-ARM HORIZONTAL ROWS

EXERCISE NOTES

- Complete the entire first tri-set two or three times before moving on to the second group of exercises.
- This is the first exercise in second tri-set of Starter Program 2.

Start

Step 1: Position and grab two cable handle attachments at shoulder height.

Step 2: *(a)* Step backward into a staggered stance so that there is tension on the cable.

Step 3: Point your palms toward the floor and keep your wrist, elbow, and shoulder on the same plane.

Midpoint

Step 4: *(b)* Pull the cables toward your shoulders, forcefully squeezing your shoulder blades together while stretching the muscles of your chest. Exhale while pulling in.

Finish

Step 5: Slowly decelerate the weight back to the starting position while feeling your back and shoulder muscles stretch (without rounding your shoulders excessively). Keep your core engaged and your legs rooted into the ground to prevent your body from being pulled forward toward the weight stack. Breathe in as the weight returns to its starting position.

Step 6: Repeat.

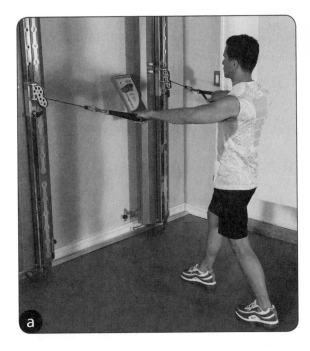
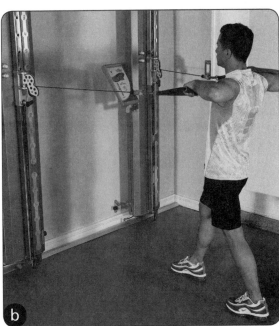

TRAINING TIP

Be careful not to rock back and forth as you pull the weight and return it to the starting position. Also, do not shrug as you pull the weights back; instead, retract your shoulder blades.

DUMBBELL WALKING LUNGES

EXERCISE NOTES

- This is the second exercise in the second tri-set of Starter Program 2.
- Complete this exercise directly after performing cable two-arm horizontal rows.

Start

Step 1: *(a)* Grab a pair of dumbbells and hold them by your sides.

Step 2: Pull your shoulder blades back and keep them retracted for the remainder of the set.

Step 3: Step forward with one leg, keeping your weight on the heel of that foot.

Midpoint

Step 4: *(b)* Sit into the hip of the front leg as you lower your back knee into a lunge.

Step 5: Continue to keep the weight on your front hip and heel as you push up through them to propel yourself back to the top.

Finish

Step 6: Step together with both feet or step forward with the back leg as you are coming to the top of your stance.

Step 7: Repeat by alternating sides.

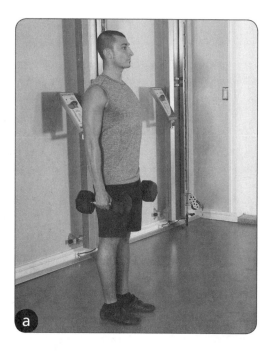 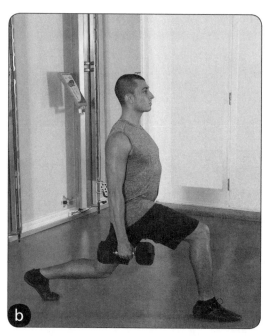

TRAINING TIP

Keep in mind that you should take a step large enough to enable you to sit into your front hip and heel without allowing your front knee to go over your toes.

DYNAMIC BRIDGING

EXERCISE NOTES

- This is the third exercise in the second tri-set of Starter Program 2.
- Complete this exercise directly after performing dumbbell walking lunges.
- Because this is the third exercise in your tri-set, you will rest after completing it.

Start

Step 1: Lie on your back.

Step 2: Pull both feet into your hips.

Step 3: Fold your arms across your chest.

Step 4: *(a)* Keep your knees directly over your ankles and your feet flat on the floor.

Step 5: Engage your glutes by squeezing them together.

Midpoint

Step 6: *(b)* Keeping your glutes engaged, exhale and push your hips off the floor as high as you can without lifting your heels.

Finish

Step 7: Slowly breathe in and lower your hips to 1 inch (2.5 cm) above the floor (do not touch).

Step 8: Repeat by lifting and lowering your hips slowly.

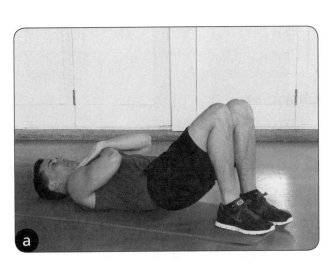

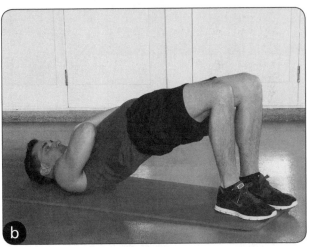

TRAINING TIP

Stay focused on using your glutes the entire time by squeezing them forcefully on the way up and allowing them to stretch on the way down. If your hamstrings cramp up, it is a sure sign that they are overactive and that your glutes aren't working hard enough!

DUMBBELL SQUAT PRESSES

EXERCISE NOTES

- Complete the dynamic warm-up exercises first.
- This is the first exercise in the second workout of Starter Program 2.

Start

Step 1: Stand with your feet shoulder-width apart holding a pair of dumbbells by your sides.

Step 2: Keep your knees bent and your core engaged throughout the set.

Step 3: Lift both dumbbells about 2 inches (5 cm) above your shoulders and face your palms away from your body.

Midpoint

Step 4: *(a)* Keep the dumbbells exactly where they are and sit back into your hips and heels into a squat (try to get parallel to the floor; use a box behind you if necessary).

Finish

Step 5: *(b)* Drive back up to a standing position through your heels and hips while simultaneously pressing the dumbbells directly overhead without rotating your wrists or arching your back.

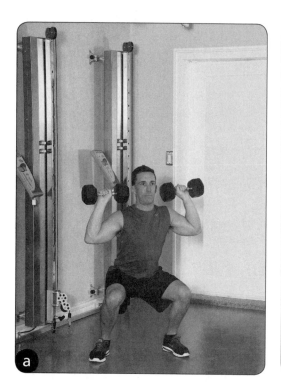
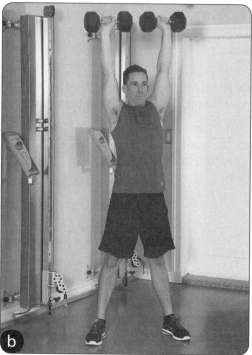

TRAINING TIP

Always sit back into your hips while squatting and remember to keep your chest up. Also, remember to breathe in on the way down and out as you're pressing the dumbbells overhead.

CHIN-UPS

EXERCISE NOTES

- This is the second exercise in the second workout of Starter Program 2.
- Complete this exercise directly after performing dumbbell squat presses.

Start

Step 1: *(a)* Grip a straight pull-up (chin-up) bar shoulder-width apart with your palms facing you.

Step 2: Engage your core to prevent swinging and then lift your legs off the floor. Crossing your legs helps provide added stability.

Midpoint

Step 3: *(b)* Use your back muscles and biceps to pull yourself up so that your chest comes up to the bar.

Finish

Step 4: Slowly lower yourself to the point right before your elbows are about to lock out.

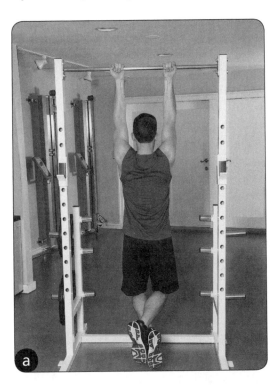
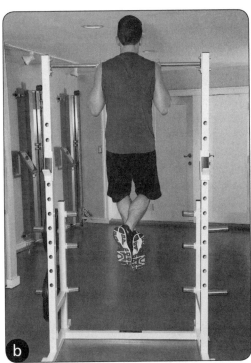

TRAINING TIP

Fight the urge to swing or to allow your elbows to lock at the bottom. Keep constant tension on your back muscles.

DUMBBELL AXE CHOPS

EXERCISE NOTES

- This is the third exercise in the second workout of Starter Program 2.
- Complete this exercise directly after performing chin-ups.
- Because this is the third exercise in your tri-set, you will rest after completing it.

Start

Step 1: Stand with your feet shoulder-width apart.

Step 2: *(a)* Hold one dumbbell above your right shoulder with your right hand on top overlapping your left.

Step 3: Engage your core before you chop and make sure to absorb the force with both your core and legs by keeping your knees bent.

Midpoint

Step 4: *(b)* Holding the weight high above your right shoulder, chop down forcefully with your arms without rotating your torso and stop abruptly right in front of your left quadriceps. Exhale while chopping.

Finish

Step 5: Breathe in and return the dumbbell to the starting position above your right shoulder.

Step 6: Repeat all repetitions on the right side and then switch to your left.

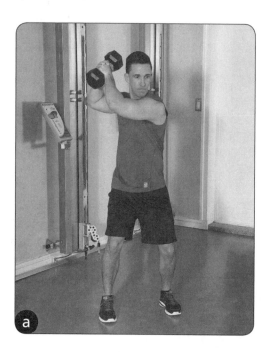 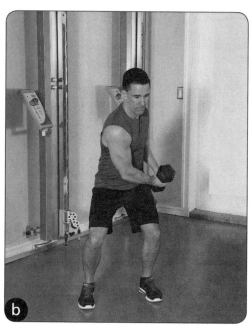

TRAINING TIP

This exercise is extremely dynamic. You can really challenge your core by chopping hard and stopping the force in an instant by tightening your core. It's an amazing exercise if you can grasp the technique with practice.

DUMBBELL ONE-LEG ROMANIAN DEADLIFTS

EXERCISE NOTES

- Complete the entire first tri-set of the second workout two or three times before moving on to the second group of exercises.
- This is the first exercise in the second tri-set of the second workout.

Start

Step 1: Grab a pair of dumbbells and hold them by your sides.

Step 2: Lift your chest up and retract your shoulder blades.

Midpoint

Step 3: *(a)* Keeping your core engaged, push back with your hips while maintaining good posture and slowly lift one leg off the floor, preparing it to stretch backward behind you.

Step 4: Allow the leg that is on the floor to stretch backward into your glutes and hamstrings while the leg that is off the floor continues to kick straight backward.

Step 5: *(b)* The dumbbells and your chest will begin to lower as your hips and free leg stretch back.

Finish

Step 6: When you can't get any deeper into your hamstring and glute stretch, do not lower your upper body. Instead, squeeze the glutes and hamstrings of the leg that is on the ground and pull your upper body back to the standing position.

Step 7: Do not allow the leg that is off the ground to touch unless you are losing balance.

Step 8: Repeat with the same leg for the specified number of repetitions, then switch to the other side.

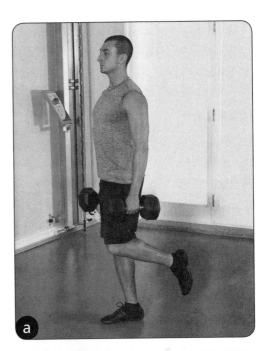

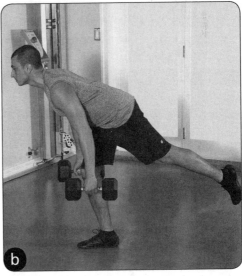

TRAINING TIP

This challenging exercise pushes your legs to the limit. Take your time and focus on balance with slightly lighter weights until you can feel your hamstrings and glutes stretching with each repetition. Remember to stay back on your heel and make sure that the foot of the leg that is off the ground points down the entire time so that you do not rotate your hips.

DIPS

EXERCISE NOTES

- This is the second exercise in the second workout of Starter Program 2.
- Complete this exercise directly after performing dumbbell one-leg Romanian deadlifts.

Start

Step 1: Using parallel bar dip handles, grip both sides and tilt your chest slightly forward.

Step 2: *(a)* Hold yourself up in the air and lift your legs off the ground.

Step 3: Keeping your elbows in alignment with your shoulders (do not allow them to spread out), slowly lower yourself down.

Midpoint

Step 4: *(b)* Stop when your biceps are parallel to the ground or just above that point if you are feeling unstable or tight through your shoulders.

Finish

Step 5: Squeeze your triceps and push yourself to the starting position.

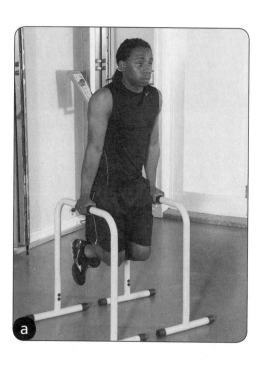 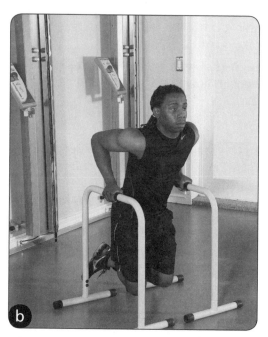

TRAINING TIP

I'm a huge fan of dips for tricep, shoulder, and chest development, but you must be careful to keep the tension on those muscles all the way through the movement. Be sure not to stretch too deep and cause too much shoulder flexion.

DUMBBELL ZOTTMAN CURLS

EXERCISE NOTES

- This is the third exercise in the second tri-set of the second workout of Starter Program 2.
- Complete this exercise directly after performing dips.
- Because this is the third exercise in your tri-set, you will rest after completing it.

Start

Step 1: (a) Stand with your feet hip-width apart and hold a pair of dumbbells by your sides.

Step 2: Keep your chest up, shoulder blades retracted, knees bent, and chin parallel to the ground throughout the set.

Step 3: (b) Moving just your forearms, rotate both dumbbells as you curl so that your palms face up. Exhale at this point to help produce more force.

Midpoint

Step 4: Squeeze your biceps forcefully without allowing your elbows to pull forward or your shoulder blades to round.

Step 5: (c) When you reach the top of your curl rotate your forearms and wrists so that your palms face the floor.

Finish

Step 6: Slowly allow the weights to lower to your legs with your palms facing down the whole way.

Step 7: Return the weights to your starting position and repeat.

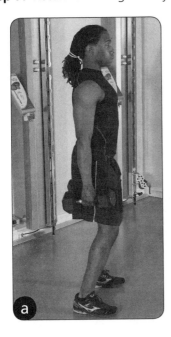 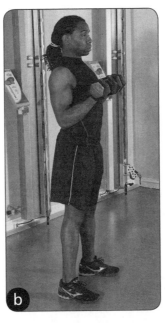 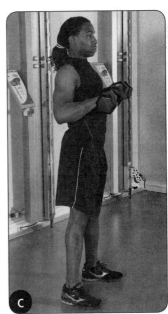

TRAINING TIP

This little known exercise challenges both your biceps and your forearms. Because it is a slightly more complex movement than a traditional dumbbell curl and uses the eccentric motion of a reverse forearm biceps curl, I suggest using a lighter weight to start—you can always go heavier later!

DECLINED PUSH-UPS

EXERCISE NOTES

- Complete the dynamic warm-up exercises first.
- This is the first exercise in the third workout of Starter Program 2.

Start

Step 1: Place both hands slightly wider than shoulder-width on the floor, positioned directly beneath your shoulders.

Step 2: *(a)* Lift your legs up and balance yourself on the balls of your feet on an elevated box, chair, bench, or step (12 to 36 inches [30 to 90 cm] high).

Step 3: Keep your core engaged and your hips level with your ankles and shoulders to form a straight diagonal line from your feet to your head.

Midpoint

Step 4: *(b)* Slowly lower your chest to just above the floor by bending your elbows and stretching your pectorals.

Finish

Step 5: Drive through your hands and push your chest back up to the starting position.

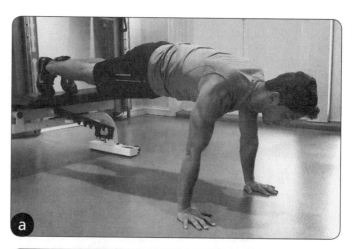

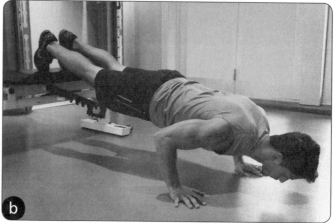

TRAINING TIP

To maximize this exercise and develop your abs and core at the same time, you should not drop your hips at all on the way down. You should even position your hips higher than parallel to your feet and shoulders to engage your core to a greater degree. Do not allow your back to arch.

DUMBBELL SHOULDER-LOADED STEP-UPS

EXERCISE NOTES

- This is the second exercise in the third workout of Starter Program 2.
- Complete this exercise directly after performing declined push-ups.

Start

Step 1: Place a box or bench on the floor in front of you that is approximately knee height.

Step 2: Hold a pair of dumbbells on your shoulders so that both heads of the dumbbells rest balanced on your shoulders. Keep your elbows lifted and pointed straight ahead of you throughout the set to keep the weights positioned correctly.

Step 3: *(a)* Place your left foot up on the step and leave your right foot on the ground.

Midpoint

Step 4: *(b)* Keep the weight on your left heel and push up through the foot and hip until you are standing up straight on top of the box.

Finish

Step 5: Keeping your right foot on the box, step down with your left leg. Do not rock backward when you land; keep your weight on the leg that is up on the box.

Step 6: Repeat by alternating legs and stepping up until you reach the desired number of repetitions.

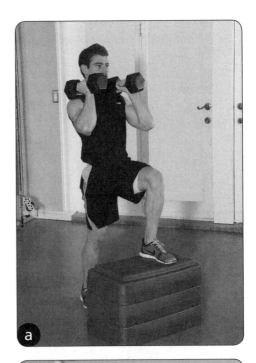

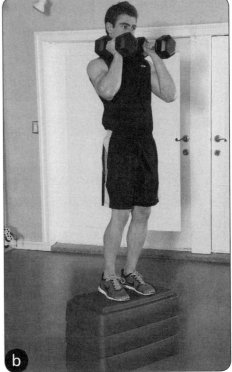

TRAINING TIP

By loading your shoulders with weight, you are engaging your core and therefore developing your midsection to a greater degree. Also, as long as you remember to keep one foot up on the box, you will not get confused by alternating legs with each rep!

BENCH LEG LIFTS

EXERCISE NOTES

- This is the third exercise in the third workout of Starter Program 2.
- Complete this exercise directly after performing dumbbell shoulder-loaded step-ups.
- Because this is the third exercise in your tri-set, you will rest after completing it.

Start

Step 1: Lie flat on your back on an exercise bench so that your hips are half on the edge of the bench and half off.

Step 2: Hold onto the bench beside your head.

Step 3: (a) Stretch your legs out straight and allow them to lower below the height of the bench until you feel a stretch through your abdomen (or before your lower back begins to arch). Keep your legs straight throughout the entire set.

Midpoint

Step 4: (b) Using your entire core, focus on contracting your abs and forcefully lifting your legs up to the point where they are positioned at a 45-degree angle.

Finish

Step 5: Slowly lower your legs back down toward the floor while keeping your core engaged. Do not arch your back.

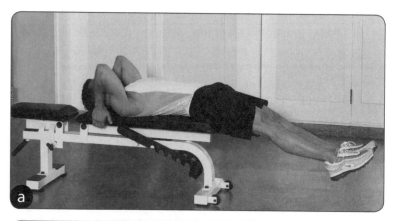

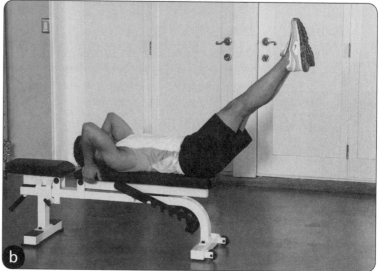

TRAINING TIP

If at first you can't lower your legs much deeper than the bench height, don't worry. After a few weeks of practice, your abs and core will be much stronger, and you will be able to stretch a little lower each week. Just make sure not to arch your back or rest at the top by bringing your legs up too high. (That's cheating!)

DUMBBELL TWO-ARM BENT-OVER ROWS

EXERCISE NOTES

- Complete the entire first tri-set of the third workout two or three times before moving on to the second group of exercises.
- This is the first exercise in second tri-set of the third workout.

Start

Step 1: Grab two dumbbells and hold them by your sides with your palms facing your body (in what is called a neutral or parallel grip).

Step 2: *(a)* Sit back with your hips into a half squat and allow your upper body to tilt forward with a neutral spine (flat back).

Midpoint

Step 3: *(b)* Holding both dumbbells beside your knees, retract your shoulder blades and pull your elbows up so that your hands reach your obliques.

Finish

Step 4: Without allowing your shoulder blades to round out, slowly lower your arms back to the starting position so that the dumbbells end beside your knees.

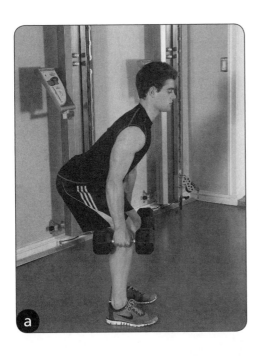
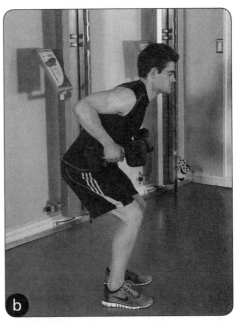

TRAINING TIP

The biggest form buster on this exercise is not sitting back in a squat and failing to remain bent over with a neutral spine throughout the movement. Your body wants to cheat and stand back up during the movement, but your stance must remain constant so that you can focus solely on squeezing your shoulder blades together as you row up.

DUMBBELL OVERHEAD SQUATS

EXERCISE NOTES

- This is the second exercise in the second tri-set of the third workout.
- Complete this exercise directly after performing dumbbell two-arm bent-over rows.

Start

Step 1: Stand with your legs shoulder-width apart.

Step 2: *(a)* Hold a dumbbell in each hand directly over your shoulders so that it looks as if you just completed a dumbbell two-arm standing shoulder press, as shown on page 66.

Step 3: Maintain excellent posture by keeping your shoulder blades back, your core engaged, and your chest up.

Midpoint

Step 4: *(b)* Keeping the weights directly above your shoulders, sit back with your hips and keep the weight on your heels as you get as deep as you can into a squat. Do not allow your knees to go over your toes or your back to round.

Finish

Step 5: Drive through your heels and glutes and push yourself back to a standing position while maintaining the same straight-arm overhead hold of the dumbbells.

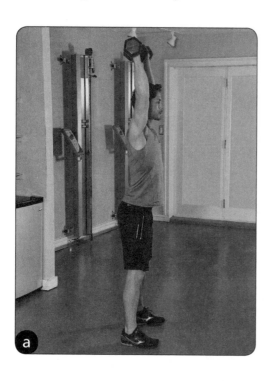 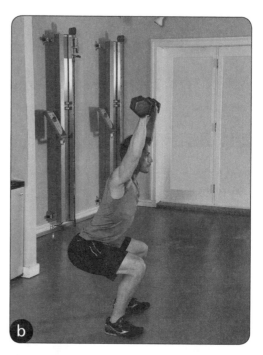

TRAINING TIP

This exercise is deceptive. Yes, it works your legs, but it's really your core that is being pushed and pulled to its limit. Start light and work on your form so that your chest doesn't collapse forward, your knees don't go over your toes, and you don't allow the dumbbells to shift forward.

MEDICINE BALL SIDE-TO-SIDE ROTATIONS

EXERCISE NOTES

- This is the third exercise in the second tri-set of Starter Program 2.
- Complete this exercise directly after performing dumbbell overhead squats.
- Because this is the third exercise in your tri-set, you will rest after completing it.

Start

Step 1: Sit down on your hips on a pad with your legs raised about 1 foot (30 cm) off the ground.

Step 2: Holding a medicine ball, look straight ahead the entire time.

Midpoint

Step 3: *(a)* Rotate your arms across your body, taking the medicine ball to the outside of your right hip.

Step 4: *(b)* Without resting the weight on your hips or on the floor, rotate the medicine ball again by taking it across your body to the outside of the other hip.

Finish

Step 5: Repeat for the desired number of reps.

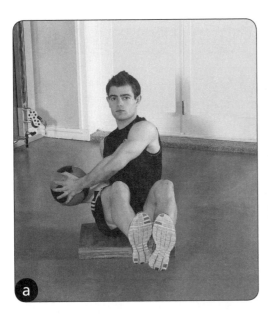
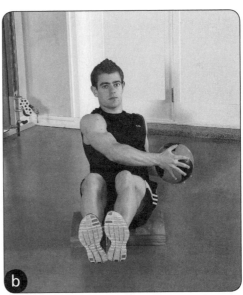

TRAINING TIP

Allow the muscles around your spine to stretch as well as resist rotation. To reduce risk of injury, do not turn your neck or twist your lower back during this movement.

CHAPTER 7

Pure Strength Workout

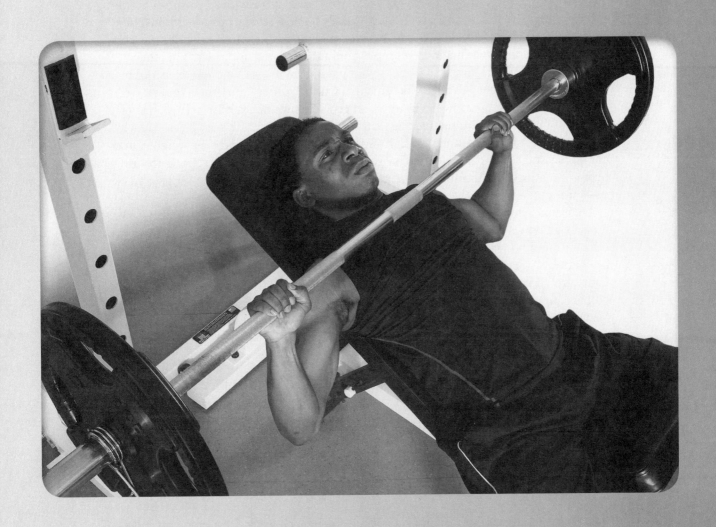

I f you've been mainly doing higher-repetition workouts, you'll be amazed at what adding in a low-rep, heavy-weight workout program can do for your body. In this workout program you'll find that your strength gains go through the roof and your muscles become denser, thicker, and harder. Of course, none of this happens by accident.

What we're going to do in the Pure Strength Workout is ditch the higher and midrange repetition schemes for a while. We're going to concentrate over the next six weeks on developing your raw strength by shooting for about five reps per set. This means that we're going to have to go heavy. You'll be lifting heavier weights than you've probably ever attempted before (with perfect form, of course). You may not even recognize yourself by week 6 as you're breaking all your previous lifting records!

The interesting part is that we're also going back to the basics. When you're lifting this heavy, you can't be fooling around on a bosu ball or concentrating on stability. We need you to have both feet firmly planted on the ground so that you can drive your feet into it as you explode with pure strength to complete each lift.

Personally, I love adding these types of programs into my periodization model throughout the year. I find that my muscles really respond to the near-maximal effort that I bring to the table each week as I perform primal compound lifts for relatively few reps. It's kind of nice having to complete only about five reps per set. This changes my mind-set and allows me to forget about pacing myself as I complete each rep.

If you haven't done a workout like this in a while (or ever), it's time to get started. Your body needs new stimulus in terms of rep schemes or exercise selection every six weeks or so. After completing the Pure Strength Workout for six weeks, you'll be able to go back to a midrange or high-repetition program, lift heavier weights, and create new personal bests because of your work throughout this strength-training program. Make sure to use table 7.1 and 7.2 and 7.3 on page 108 as a basis to track your workouts.

I have just a few words of caution for you. We're going to be going heavy here, but that doesn't mean that you should ever attempt a lift that you don't feel comfortable with. Maintain form with each rep and remember that when your form begins to break down, the set is over, even if you didn't reach the number of repetitions that you were shooting for. We're in this weightlifting game for the long run, so keep your head in the game, lift smart, and go heavy!

Now let's talk about the top 10 tips that I want you to remember during this program.

Top 10 Tips and Benefits of the Pure Strength Workout:

1. You're going to create a ton of new personal bests for your lifts!

2. The simple, compound movements allow you to go heavy.

3. Instead of using tri-sets we'll be using opposing-exercise supersets (two exercises done back to back) to allow you to recover faster between sets.

4. The intensity of the exercise will come from the heavy weight that you are lifting. Therefore, you'll still find yourself huffing and puffing after each round of exercises.

5. Be sure to time your rest and keep it consistent each week. Less rest won't allow you to lift as much weight, and added rest will allow you to go even heavier. Just keep it between two and three minutes between supersets.

6. Take about 20 to 30 seconds between exercises in your superset to grab the weights that you'll need, and get yourself in position.

7. During your first week of this program, you should do one less set per exercise and not focus on lifting your heaviest weights possible. Instead, you should focus on your form and technique.

8. I love lifting heavy as much as the next guy, but don't try to be a hero and blow out your back by neglecting proper form. Don't be that guy.

9. As always, you're probably not going to feel comfortable doing one or two of these new exercises but remember that those are the ones that you most likely need the most. Start out slow and light until you master the form. Gradually increase the resistance each week. You'll be surprised at what you can accomplish in just six weeks!

10. By the end of the Pure Strength Workout program, you'll have a stronger body that is made up of denser and firmer muscles. Every time you're trying to muster up the mental and physical energy to complete your next set, think of all the benefits that the program is creating for you!

Table 7.1   Pure Strength Workout, Workout Chart 1

Exercise	Sets	Reps	Tempo	Week 1	Week 2	Week 3	Week 4	Week 5	Week 6
W1. Split jacks	1	30–60 s	1-1-1-1	Weights					
W2. Transverse plane lunges	1	20	2-1-1-0						
W3. Hand walkouts	1	10	1-1-1-1						
(Once warm-up exercises are completed, begin strength training.)									
1A. Dumbbell flat chest presses	5	5	3-0-1-1						
1B. Barbell back squats	5	5	3-0-1-1						
(Rest 2–3 minutes and repeat exercises 1A and 1B.)									
2A. Barbell bent-over rows	5	5	2-0-1-1						
2B. Barbell Romanian deadlifts	5	5	3-0-1-1						
(Rest 2–3 minutes and repeat exercises 2A and 2B.)									

Table 7.2 Pure Strength Workout, Workout Chart 2

Exercise	Sets	Reps	Tempo	Week 1	Week 2	Week 3	Week 4	Week 5	Week 6
W1. Split jacks	1	30–60 s	1-1-1-1	Weights					
W2. Transverse plane lunges	1	20	2-1-1-0						
W3. Hand walkouts	1	10	1-1-1-1						
(Once warm-up exercises are completed, begin strength training.)									
1A. Barbell military shoulder presses	4	8-5	2-0-1-1						
1B. Dumbbell deadlifts with pronated grip	4	8-5	3-0-1-1						
(Rest 2–3 minutes and repeat exercises 1A and 1B.)									
2A. Pull-ups (weighted)	4	8-5	2-0-1-1						
2B. Barbell split lunges	4	2 × 8-5	3-0-1-1						
(Rest 2–3 minutes and repeat exercises 2A and 2B.)									

Table 7.3 Pure Strength Workout, Workout Chart 3

Exercise	Sets	Reps	Tempo	Week 1	Week 2	Week 3	Week 4	Week 5	Week 6
W1. Split jacks	1	30–60 s	1-1-1-1	Weights					
W2. Transverse plane lunges	1	20	2-1-1-0						
W3. Hand walkouts	1	10	1-1-1-1						
(Once warm-up exercises are completed, begin strength training.)									
1A. Barbell incline chest presses	5	5	3-0-1-1						
1B. Dumbbell one-leg step-ups	5	2 × 5	1-0-1-1						
(Rest 2–3 minutes and repeat exercises 1A and 1B.)									
2A. Cable seated rows	4	8-5	2-0-1-1						
2B. Barbell front squats	4	8-5	3-0-1-1						
(Rest 2–3 minutes and repeat exercises 2A and 2B.)									

SPLIT JACKS

EXERCISE NOTES

Complete the dynamic warm-up exercises before performing all three weight workouts in the Pure Strength Workout.

Start

Step 1: Stand with your legs hip-width apart and your hands by your sides.

Step 2: *(a)* Step out with your left foot and raise your right arm in the air above your shoulder.

Step 3: Tighten your core and lean slightly forward.

Midpoint

Step 4: *(b)* Quickly jump and switch legs and arms at the same time, landing on the balls of your feet.

Finish

Step 5: Repeat this motion by rapidly switching the front leg and arm with the back ones for 30 to 60 seconds.

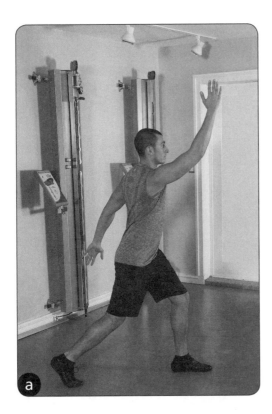
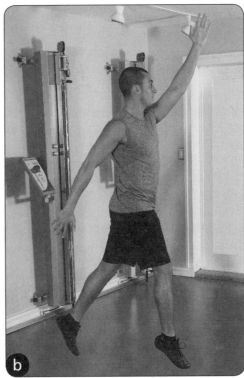

TRAINING TIP

Try to think of this exercise as doing jumping jacks in the sagittal plane by jumping forward and back instead of side to side (frontal plane). Concentrate on landing softly and absorbing impact so that your joints stay safe.

TRANSVERSE PLANE LUNGES

EXERCISE NOTES

- Complete the dynamic warm-up exercises first before performing all three weight workouts in the Pure Strength Workout.
- Complete this exercise directly after performing split jacks.

Start

Step 1: *(a)* Stand with your feet together. Clench your fists and raise your arms so that your hands are at shoulder level.

Step 2: Think of yourself as standing on the twelve o'clock position on a clock. *(b)* Then take a big step to your right side so that you land at three o'clock. (Your right foot will now be turned out at a right angle approximately facing the three o'clock position perpendicular to your left leg, which remains at twelve o'clock.)

Midpoint

Step 3: Absorb the landing of your right foot by keeping the weight back into your heel and decelerating into your right hip.

Step 4: Do not allow your right knee to go over the toes of your right foot; keep sitting back into your hips. Also, straighten your left leg fully and feel the stretch on the inner thigh of that leg.

Finish

Step 5: Push through your right hip and heel and accelerate back to the starting position, bringing both feet together and standing up straight so that both feet are standing on the twelve o'clock position facing forward.

Step 6: Repeat the same technique on the opposite side by lunging with your left leg onto the nine o'clock position. Your left leg will now be bent, and your right will be straight.

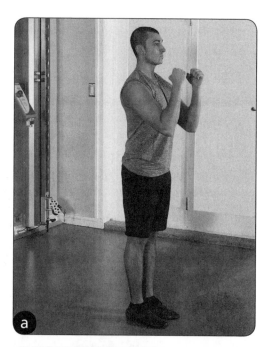

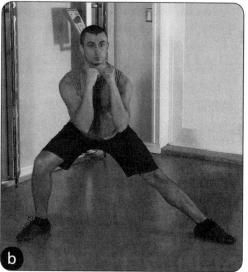

TRAINING TIP

Although this exercise works to open up your hips by using the rotational plane of motion, make sure that you do not overtwist your upper torso, which should remain square with your hips throughout the set.

HAND WALKOUTS

EXERCISE NOTES

- Complete the dynamic warm-up exercises first before performing all three weight workouts in the Pure Strength Workout.
- Complete this exercise directly after performing transverse plane lunges.

Start

Step 1: Stand with your feet slightly apart.

Step 2: *(a)* Place both hands directly on the floor in front of your feet.

Step 3: Keep your fingers and palms in contact with the ground throughout the set and begin walking your hands out, one after the other.

Midpoint

Step 4: *(b)* Make sure to keep your core engaged the entire time so that you do not let your hips drop toward the floor. Walk your hands out past the push-up position if possible and stay on the balls of your feet.

Finish

Step 5: Begin to walk your hands back to the starting position while allowing your hips to rise up in the air. Stop when you cannot stretch any farther into your hamstrings, glutes, or calves, or if your palms begin to come off the floor.

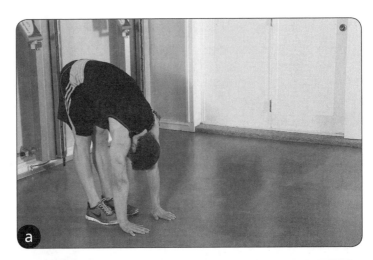

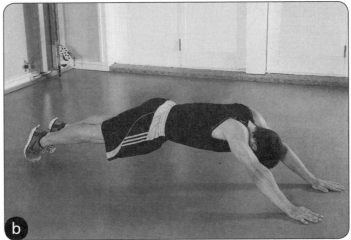

TRAINING TIP

This warm-up is one of my favorite ways to get the core, shoulder complex, and arms fired up for the workout. It has the added benefit of stretching tight calves, hamstrings, glutes, and the lower back!

DUMBBELL FLAT CHEST PRESSES

EXERCISE NOTES

- Complete the dynamic warm-up exercises first.
- This is the first exercise in the first workout of the Pure Strength Workout.

Start

Step 1: Sit on a bench holding two dumbbells on the tops of your thighs.

Step 2: Lie backward and kick the dumbbells back one at a time until they rest on your chest.

Step 3: *(a)* Rotate your palms away from you so that the heads of the dumbbells are directly above your chest and shoulders.

Midpoint

Step 4: *(b)* Squeeze your pectoral muscles, press the weights directly over your chest, and allow the dumbbells to come together in an arc, but do not bang them against each other at the top.

Finish

Step 5: Slowly decelerate the weights back to the starting position while feeling your chest and shoulder muscles stretch. Keep the tension on your chest the entire time and maintain stability in your shoulder joints. You should aim to take the weights down about 1 inch (2.5 cm) above your shoulders and chest but do not go so deep that you lose tension on your chest and place the stress on the connective tissue of your shoulder joints instead.

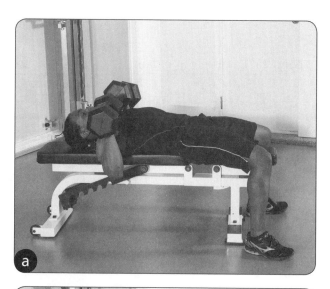

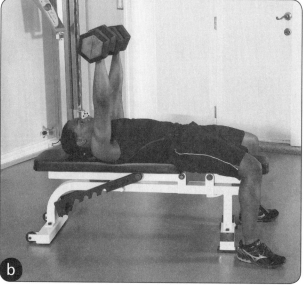

TRAINING TIP

I prefer using dumbbells for the flat bench press instead of a barbell because there is less stress on your shoulder joints. By using dumbbells you allow your arms and shoulders to rotate externally into a more natural position, which alleviates a lot of the shoulder injuries and issues typically associated with benching.

BARBELL BACK SQUATS

EXERCISE NOTES

- This is the second exercise in the Pure Strength Workout.
- Complete this exercise directly after performing dumbbell flat chest presses.

Start

Step 1: Stand with your feet shoulder-width apart and place a slight bend in your knees.

Step 2: *(a)* Step under the barbell and place it directly on your trapezius muscles below your neck. Hold the bar just outside shoulder-width apart.

Step 3: Maintain a flat back (neutral spine) and retract your shoulder blades for posture throughout the set. Also, make sure to keep your chest up and your chin parallel to the floor.

Midpoint

Step 4: *(b)* Slowly breathe in and sit back with your hips, keeping the weight on your heels. Get as deep as you can without rounding out your lower back, letting your heels come up, dropping your chest, or going into a posterior pelvic tilt.

Finish

Step 5: Push as hard you can through your hips and heels, propelling yourself back to the standing start position.

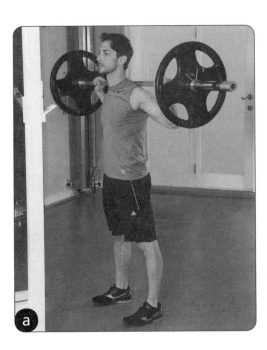 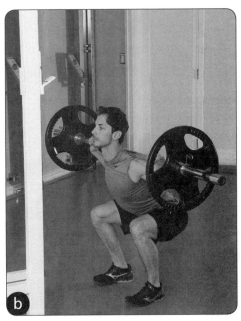

TRAINING TIP

The great thing about doing the barbell back squat as the first leg exercise in this program to start the week is that you will be able to lift your heaviest weights and therefore reap the most benefit. If you remember to keep your form tight, you will see massive strength and size gains in a matter of weeks!

BARBELL BENT-OVER ROWS

EXERCISE NOTES

- Complete the entire first superset three or four times before moving on to the second group of exercises in the first workout.
- This is the first exercise in the second superset of the Pure Strength Workout.

Start

Step 1: Stand over a barbell with your feet about shoulder-width apart and grip the bar slightly wider than your thighs using an overhand pronated grip.

Step 2: Using a tight grip, tight core, and neutral spine, pull the bar off the rack and allow it to rest against your quads as you stand up straight.

Step 3: Sit back with your hips into a half squat and allow your upper body to tilt forward with a neutral spine (flat back) until you reach about a 45-degree angle.

Midpoint

Step 4: *(a)* Holding the bar right in front of your knees, *(b)* retract your shoulder blades and pull your elbows up so that the bar pulls into your abs.

Finish

Step 5: Without allowing your shoulder blades to round out, slowly lower the bar back to the starting position so that the barbell comes right in front of your knees.

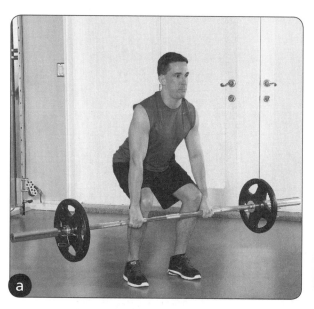 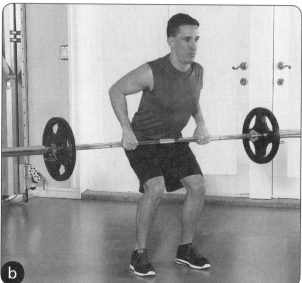

TRAINING TIP

Besides not allowing your back to round or yourself to stand up as you row the weight, focus on not shrugging the weight with your traps and allowing your elbows to flare out to the sides. Instead, keep your elbows close to your body and stay down in your stance so that you can retract your shoulder blades and use your big back muscles to move the weight.

BARBELL ROMANIAN DEADLIFTS

EXERCISE NOTES

- This is the second exercise in the second superset of the first workout of the Pure Strength Workout.
- Complete this exercise directly after performing barbell bent-over rows.
- Because this is the second exercise in your superset, you will rest after completing it.

Start

Step 1: Stand over a barbell with your feet hip-width apart and grip the bar slightly wider than your thighs using an overhand alternate grip (one hand palm facing up and the other palm facing down).

Step 2: *(a)* Maintaining a tight grip, tight core, and neutral spine, pull the bar off the rack and allow it to rest against your quads. Keeping a flat back (neutral spine), retract your shoulder blades and place a slight bend in your knees.

Midpoint

Step 3: *(b)* Allow your hips to stretch backward (with as much as a 20-degree bend in your knees) until you can't stretch your hamstrings and glutes anymore. Your upper body will lower a little, but the hips always move first and dictate how low you go. Do not drop your upper torso toward the floor as you lower the weight just to get deeper into the movement. This action will not provide any more benefit to your legs and may lead to injury.

Finish

Step 4: Squeeze your glutes, push your hips forward, and pull your upper body back to the starting position before performing the next repetition. Exhale as you exert force and lift up.

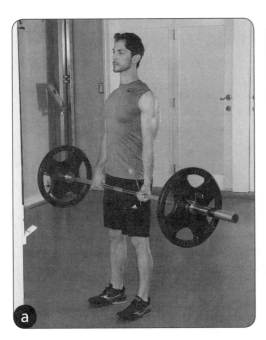
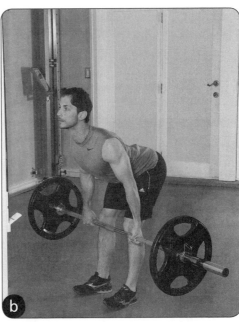

TRAINING TIP

Keep your weight back on your heels and make sure to end the movement when your hips will not stretch back behind you any farther.

BARBELL MILITARY SHOULDER PRESSES

EXERCISE NOTES

- Complete the dynamic warm-up exercises first.
- This is the first exercise in the second workout of the Pure Strength Workout.

Start

Step 1: *(a)* Stand with your feet shoulder-width apart and hold a barbell with your palms facing away from you in a grip slightly wider than shoulder-width apart. The barbell should be at, or just above, your shoulders.

Step 2: Keep your knees bent and your core engaged throughout the set.

Midpoint

Step 3: *(b)* Press the barbell directly overhead without arching your lower back or tilting your head too far back.

Finish

Step 4: Slowly decelerate the weight back to the starting position above your shoulders while keeping tension on the deltoids.

Step 5: Maintain form and repeat.

TRAINING TIP

This exercise is a fantastic mass builder for your shoulders, so you'll want to load up the bar with as much weight as you can handle with good form. But be conscious throughout the set about not arching your lower back and make sure that you can decelerate the weight back down to the starting position after you lift it overhead.

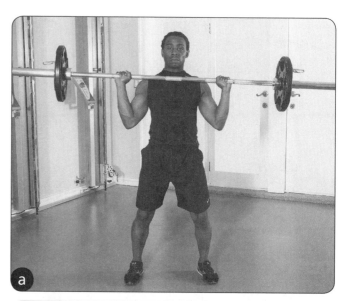

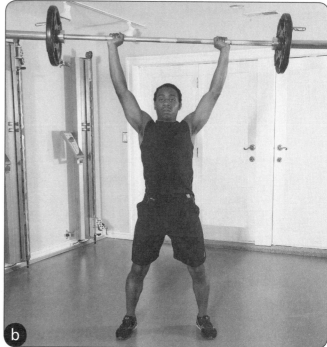

DUMBBELL DEADLIFTS WITH PRONATED GRIP

EXERCISE NOTES

- This is the second exercise in the second workout of the Pure Strength Workout.
- Complete this exercise directly after performing barbell military shoulder presses.
- Because this is the second exercise in your superset, you will rest after completing it.

Start

Step 1: Grab a pair of dumbbells and hold them by your sides.

Step 2: *(a)* Rotate the dumbbells so that they rest against your quadriceps with your palms facing your body (your palms will remain facing your body throughout the set).

Step 3: Lift your chest up and retract your shoulder blades.

Midpoint

Step 4: Keeping your core engaged, sit back with your hips while maintaining good posture and keeping your weight on your heels.

Step 5: *(b)* Slowly sit back with your hips as deep as you can into a squat position so that your upper legs are approximately parallel to the floor (make sure to stop before your hips and lower back round out).

Finish

Step 6: Drive through your heels, pull your chest up while exhaling, and push your body back to a standing position.

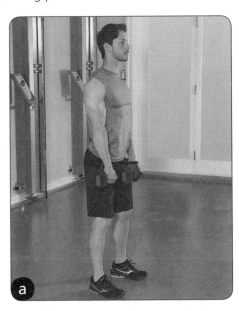
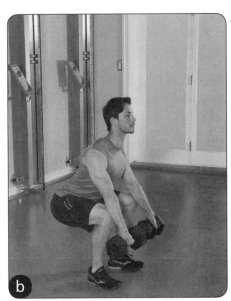

TRAINING TIP

Although I think that the barbell deadlift is a terrific exercise, the truth is that most people are far too tight through their hamstrings, quadratus lumborum (lower back area), and hips to do it safely. I've seen too many guys tweak the lower back trying to pull a heavy barbell deadlift from the floor. That's why I suggest using dumbbells to mimic the movement while getting as deep as you can until you improve your flexibility over time.

PULL-UPS (WEIGHTED)

EXERCISE NOTES

- Complete the entire first superset three or four times before moving on to the second group of exercises.
- This is the first exercise in the second superset of the second workout of the Pure Strength Workout.

Start

Step 1: Grip a straight pull-up (chin-up) bar with your hands shoulder-width apart and your palms facing away from you. Wear a weight belt with a weight plate attached for resistance.

Step 2: *(a)* Engage your core to prevent yourself from swinging and then lift your legs off the floor by bending your knees. Crossing your legs can improve stability.

Midpoint

Step 3: *(b)* Using your back, biceps, and forearm muscles, pull yourself up so that your chest comes up to the bar and your forearms touch your biceps.

Finish

Step 4: Slowly lower yourself to the point just before your elbows lock out.

Step 5: Repeat and add weight if necessary to increase the difficulty of the exercise so that you can achieve the desired repetition range. You can use a weighted vest, wear a weighted belt, or hold a dumbbell between your feet for added resistance.

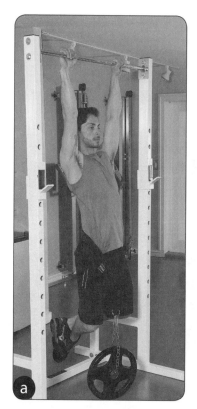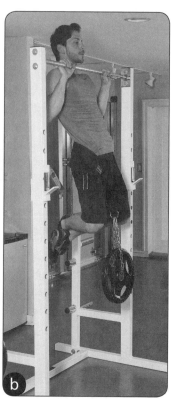

TRAINING TIP

Pull-ups may be the absolute best back exercise for creating that V shape that all guys are aiming for. This V shape (your lats) makes your waist look smaller and your shoulders broader. My tip to improve your results with pull-ups is to use a full range of motion. Use a band for assistance in the beginning if you need to. Then, as you gradually build up strength, you will be able to switch over to unassisted pull-ups.

BARBELL SPLIT LUNGES

EXERCISE NOTES

- This is the second exercise in the second superset of the second workout of the Pure Strength Workout.
- Complete this exercise directly after performing pull-ups (weighted).
- Because this is the second exercise in your superset, you will rest after completing it.

Start

Step 1: Position yourself under a squat rack and place a barbell along your trapezius muscles as you would for a barbell back squat.

Step 2: Keep your chest up, shoulder blades retracted, and chin parallel to the ground throughout the set.

Step 3: *(a)* Pick the bar off the squat rack and step back with one leg (keep this leg back for all 8-5 reps).

Midpoint

Step 4: Keeping your chest up, slowly bend and lower the knee of your back leg toward the floor as you keep the weight on your front hip and heel.

Step 5: *(b)* When you reach the bottom (about 2 inches [5 cm] above the floor), you should feel a stretch through your back quadriceps and hip flexors and have most of the weight on the front hip and heel. Your legs should approximately form two right angles (or slightly wider).

Finish

Step 6: Quickly push through your front hip and the heel of the front foot to raise yourself up to the starting position.

Step 7: Repeat with the same leg and then switch sides before returning the barbell to the rack.

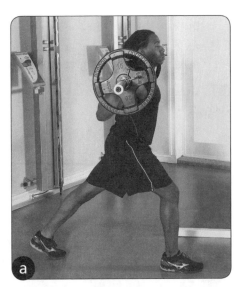

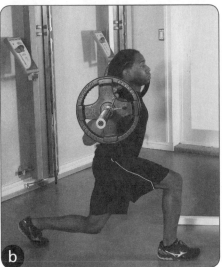

TRAINING TIP

This exercise is also referred to as a split squat, but because it is really a lunging movement that is what I will call it to reduce the confusion between movements (I call a lunge a lunge and a squat a squat). The biggest difficulty that guys have with this exercise is that they tilt forward with the upper body on the way down and, because of tight quads, sometimes can't stretch very far down with the back leg. By starting lighter and working on form, core strength, and hip flexor and quad flexibility, you will master this exercise in no time!

BARBELL INCLINE CHEST PRESSES

EXERCISE NOTES

- Complete the dynamic warm-up exercises first.
- This is the first exercise in the third workout of the Pure Strength Workout.

Start

Step 1: Lie back on a 45-degree incline bench directly under a barbell and have both feet firmly planted on the floor.

Step 2: *(a)* Grip the bar just outside shoulder-width apart and lift it off the bench press rack, holding it directly above your chest.

Midpoint

Step 3: *(b)* Lower the barbell down slowly toward the top of your chest. The bar should stop 1 to 2 inches (2.5 to 5 cm) above your chest.

Finish

Step 4: To help produce force, exhale as you press the bar above your chest to return it to the starting position.

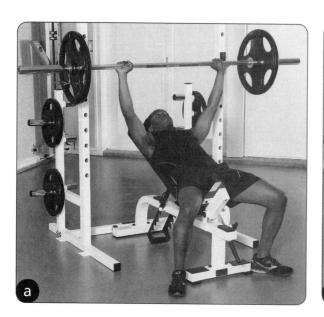
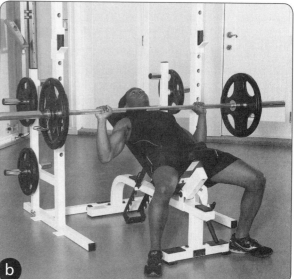

TRAINING TIP

This exercise helps you build up the area between your shoulders and chest to create a fuller looking, more muscular chest. Remember to keep your feet, back, and head in a five-point position at all times.

DUMBBELL ONE-LEG STEP-UPS

EXERCISE NOTES

- This is the second exercise in the third workout of the Pure Strength Workout.
- Complete this exercise directly after performing barbell incline chest presses.
- Because this is the second exercise in your superset, you will rest after completing it.

Start

Step 1: Place a box or bench of about knee height on the floor in front of you.

Step 2: Hold a pair of heavy dumbbells by your sides with a tight neutral grip. Ensure that your posture remains strong by keeping your shoulder blades pulled back while lifting your chest up.

Step 3: *(a)* Place your left foot up on the step and leave your right foot on the ground.

Midpoint

Step 4: *(b)* Keep the weight on your left heel and push up through the foot and hip until you are standing up straight on top of the box.

Finish

Step 5: Continue to keep your left foot on the box and step back down slowly. Your right foot should absorb the impact so that you can barely hear that foot land. Do not rock backward when you land and keep the weight on the hip and heel of the left leg throughout the set.

Step 6: Complete five repetitions with the left leg and then switch to the right.

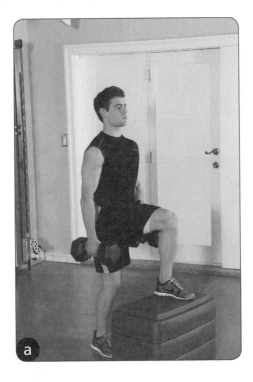 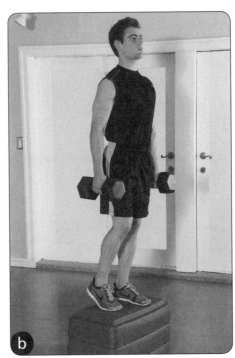

TRAINING TIP

Do not underestimate the power of this simple step-up exercise. If you use enough weight you will create stronger, more muscular legs, and your heart will be pounding by the end of the set!

CABLE SEATED ROWS

EXERCISE NOTES

- Complete the entire first superset three or four times before moving on to the second group of exercises.
- This is the first exercise in the second superset of the third workout of the Pure Strength Workout.

Start

Step 1: Attach a close-grip handle to a seated row machine or cable machine with a bench and grip it using a neutral or parallel grip while seated on the bench of the machine.

Step 2: *(a)* With your knees bent, place both feet against the footrest of the machine, grab the handle, engage your core, and retract your shoulder blades.

Step 3: Push back with both legs to keep your starting position while maintaining a neutral spine and good posture. Ensure that you have a small bend in your knees throughout the set.

Midpoint

Step 4: *(b)* Concentrate on squeezing your shoulder blades back while stretching open your chest as you complete your first repetition, pulling the handle of the cable into your abdomen.

Finish

Step 5: Without allowing your shoulder blades or back to round excessively forward, return your arms to their extended starting position. Maintain tension on your back muscles at all times.

Step 6: Repeat for the desired number of reps.

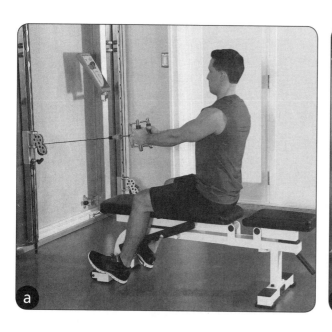
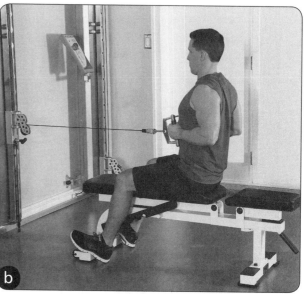

TRAINING TIP

Although many guys love this exercise, it can turn ugly real fast when you lean all the way back as you row the weight or round all the way forward as you return the weight to its starting position. Stick with proper form and you'll enjoy a healthy back and better gains too!

BARBELL FRONT SQUATS

EXERCISE NOTES

- This is the second exercise in the second superset of the third workout of the Pure Strength Workout.
- Complete this exercise directly after performing cable seated rows.
- Because this is the second exercise in your superset, you will rest after completing it.

Start

Step 1: Stand with your feet hip-width apart and your knees slightly bent.

Step 2: *(a)* Step under the barbell and place it directly on your anterior deltoid and other shoulder muscles. The bar should touch the front of your neck right above your collarbone. (The bar is in the right position if you can balance it without touching it with your hands.)

Step 3: Grab the bar by folding your arms over it and holding it with your hands face down. Alternatively, you can use a traditional front squat grip by rotating your elbows forward, allowing your fingers and wrists to stretch back, and resting your palms on top of your shoulders while balancing the bar.

Midpoint

Step 4: Slowly breathe in, keep your chest and elbows lifted high, and sit back with your hips, keeping the weight on your heels.

Step 5: *(b)* Squat as deep as you can without rounding out your lower back, letting your heels come up, allowing your knees to go over your toes, dropping your chest, or going into a posterior pelvic tilt.

Finish

Step 6: Drive hard through your hips and heels to propel yourself back to the standing start position.

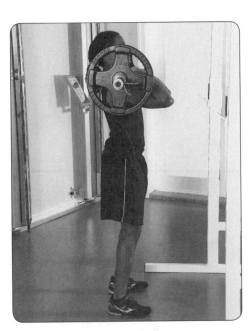

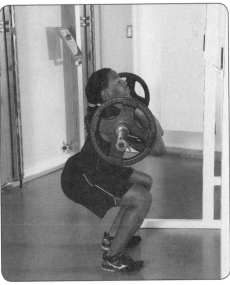

TRAINING TIP

You don't see the average guy doing this exercise for a reason—it's hard! But if you can get over the fact that you won't be able to front squat as much as you back squat, you'll be way ahead of the game. This exercise is phenomenal for developing a powerful core (abs) and massive quads!

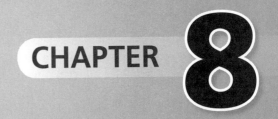

Chapter 8

Core Power Workout

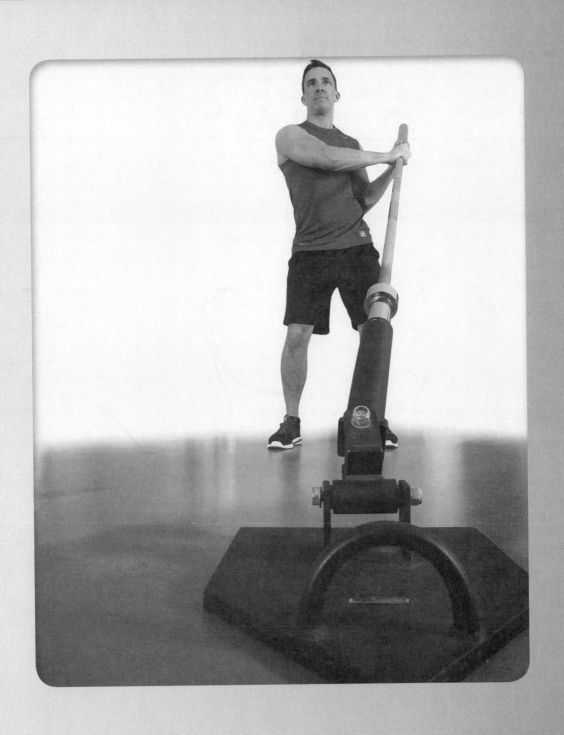

I can remember a few years back when the latest fitness craze was standing on a bosu ball with one leg raised in the air while juggling a pair of dumbbells. Well, maybe the whole functional core training fad didn't take it quite that far, but I did occasionally see trainers having their clients do things that left me scratching my head.

For example, although training on an unstable surface can be useful, rarely is there a good reason to jump up on a stability ball and try to do two dozen squats. That exercise would carry a high risk and produce few benefits in terms of strengthening your core or legs when considering a risk/benefit ratio.

A better choice would be to pick functional core-based exercises based on their movement patterns. By doing this, you will ensure that you're targeting every muscle in your core to strengthen and tighten the entire area.

Your core consists of many muscles and muscle groups that work to stabilize your spine, shoulder girdle, and pelvis when flexed. Although your core is defined in various ways depending on the source, it typically includes the muscles of your torso, hips, and neck—basically everything but your limbs and head.

By having a strong core you are better able to stabilize your body and provide a strong foundation on which to fire explosive energy to your limbs. This energy yields amazing force and speed when used in the gym or on the playing field. For that reason, training your core is crucial.

I've designed a four- to six-week program that you can use to strengthen your back, abs, obliques, and every other core muscle in your body. The result will be a stronger back, a tighter waistline, and better-looking abs that you can feel good about showing off when you remove your shirt.

I've designed this workout to include three distinct types of training stimuli to maximize your efforts while in the gym. You'll be going through a strength and power day, a hypertrophy workout, and a high-intensity circuit. This program is just plain fun to do!

Unless your main goal is bodybuilding, you'll enjoy the four to six weeks off from bench pressing, lat pull-downs, and heavy squats. You'll have plenty of time to get back into those important movements again, but this Core Power Workout will provide your body with some much needed periodized time off from those exercises. The three workouts will also help to mold you into a more well-rounded athlete. Make sure to use table 8.1 and tables 8.2 and 8.3 on page 128 as a basis to track your workouts.

OK, we've talked enough about how much fun you're going to have digging into this program or how much tighter your midsection will be after completing the Core Power Workout. Let's talk about the top 10 tips that I want you to remember before we jump into the routine.

Top 10 Tips and Benefits of the Core Power Workout:

1. This routine will be a shock to your system if you've been concentrating on bench presses, pull-downs, and heavy leg exercises. This means that you'll wake up muscles that you haven't used in this way in years. The routine will help you become even stronger when you decide to go back to your heavier lifts.

2. Because this routine involves more than just strength-based exercises, you can choose to switch it up after four weeks if you plateau before the sixth week.

3. You'll find three distinct workouts to help maximize core strength and power!

4. Because each workout includes different repetition and set variations, read the recommended sets and reps for each day carefully.

5. Although you won't be benching extremely heavy weights, you still need to bring your A game. Pick up the intensity each week and train hard!

6. Remember to engage your core by flexing your abs (not drawing in) before each movement to stabilize your spine and hips.

7. If a movement is new to you, be sure to ease into it with a lighter weight (or your body weight) until you master the form.

8. Begin to view great-looking abs as more than just decoration for your midsection. Your core is your energy center and should be as functional as it looks.

9. After four to six weeks of consistent Core Power Workouts, you will find that you are stronger when you get back into your more traditional heavy presses and pulls because you'll be better able to stabilize your core and produce more force.

10. Completing the Core Power Workout will strengthen and tighten your midsection better than all the crunches in the world, and it's healthier for your back as well!

Table 8.1   Core Power Workout, Workout Chart 1

Exercise	Sets	Reps	Tempo	Week 1	Week 2	Week 3	Week 4	Week 5	Week 6
W1. Squat thrusts (burpees)	1	10	1-1-1-1	Weights					
W2. Curtsy lunges	1	2 × 12	2-1-1-1						
W3. Planks with shoulder abduction	1	20	1-1-1-1						
(Once warm-up exercises are completed, begin strength training.)									
1A. Barbell push presses	5	5	2-0-1-1						
1B. Barbell front squats	5	5	3-0-1-1						
(Rest 2–3 minutes and repeat exercises 1A and 1B.)									
2A. Dumbbell one-leg reach to rows	4	8-5	2-0-1-1						
2B. Barbell combat twists	4	16	1-0-1-0						
(Rest 2–3 minutes and repeat exercises 2A and 2B.)									
3A. Cable kneeling rope chops	2–3	2 × 10-12	2-0-1-1						
(Rest 60 to 90 s and repeat exercise 3A.)									

Table 8.2 Core Power Workout, Workout Chart 2

Exercise	Sets	Reps	Tempo	Week 1	Week 2	Week 3	Week 4	Week 5	Week 6
W1. Squat thrusts (burpees)	1	10	1-1-1-1	Weights					
W2. Curtsey lunges	1	2 × 12	2-1-1-1						
W3. Plank with shoulder abduction	1	20	1-1-1-1						
(Once warm-up exercises are completed, begin strength training.)									
1A. T-twist push-ups	3	16-20	1-0-1-1						
1B. Barbell one-leg good mornings	3	2 × 12-10	3-0-1-1						
1C. Stability ball roll-outs	3	12-15	2-0-1-0						
(Rest 90 s and repeat exercises 1A, 1B, and 1C.)									
2A. Dumbbell one-arm prone rows	3	2 × 12	3-0-1-1						
2B. Barbell overhead squats	3	12-10	3-0-1-1						
2C. Unilateral bird dogs	3	2 × 10	1-0-1-1						
(Rest 90 s and repeat exercises 2A, 2B, and 2C.)									

Table 8.3 Core Power Workout, Workout Chart 3

Exercise	Sets	Reps	Tempo	Week 1	Week 2	Week 3	Week 4	Week 5	Week 6
W1. Squat thrusts (burpees)	1	10	1-1-1-1	Weights					
W2. Curtsy lunges	1	2 × 12	2-1-1-1						
W3. Plank with shoulder abduction	1	20	1-1-1-1						
(Once warm-up exercises are completed, begin strength training.)									
1A. Cable low to high rope chops	3–4	2 × 12	1-0-1-1						
1B. Medicine ball slams	3–4	15	1-0-1-0						
1C. Side planks with reach under	3–4	2 × 15	1-1-1-1						
1D. Dumbbell walking lunges with chop	3–4	20	2-1-1-0						
1E. Cobras	3–4	12-15	1-0-1-1						
(Rest 2–3 minutes and repeat exercises 1A, 1B, 1C, 1D, and 1E.)									

SQUAT THRUSTS (BURPEES)

EXERCISE NOTES

Complete the dynamic warm-up exercises first before performing all three weight workouts in the Core Power Workout.

Start

Step 1: *(a)* Stand with your legs hip-width apart and your arms raised overhead.

Step 2: Bend over and place your hands on the floor about shoulder-width apart in front of your feet.

Step 3: *(b)* Jump back with both legs and land in a push-up position (engage your core and do not let your hips sag down toward the floor).

Midpoint

Step 4: *(c)* Complete a push-up.

Finish

Step 5: From the top of your push-up position, jump both legs back up to your hands.

Step 6: Stand back up straight and raise your arms over your head.

Step 7: Repeat up to 10 times.

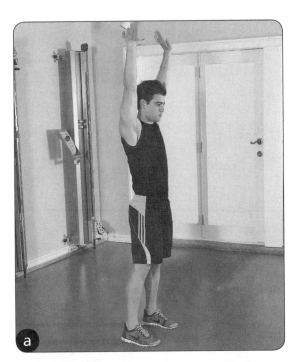

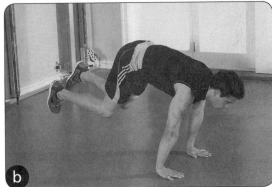

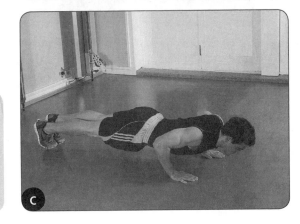

TRAINING TIP

If you are concerned about your form or joints when you are asked to jump back and jump in, I recommend placing one foot back (or in) at a time to minimize the force on your joints. Concentrate on landing softly and absorbing the impact.

CURTSY LUNGES

EXERCISE NOTES

- Complete the dynamic warm-up exercises before performing all three weight workouts in the Core Power Workout.
- Complete this exercise directly after performing squat thrusts (burpees).

Start

Step 1: *(a)* Stand with your legs hip-width apart and your arms held at your sides.

Step 2: Keep your chest raised up high and step back approximately 2 feet (60 cm) with your right foot so that it lands behind you and to the outside of your left foot.

Midpoint

Step 3: *(b)* Sit back into your left hip and allow your back (right) knee to decelerate slowly down to 3 to 4 inches (8 or 10 cm) above the floor.

Finish

Step 4: Push back up to your starting position using your left hip and heel to produce force.

Step 5: Stand up straight and perform all repetitions with your right leg lunging back before moving to your left leg.

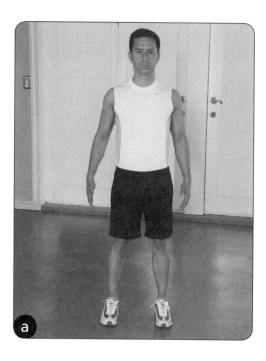 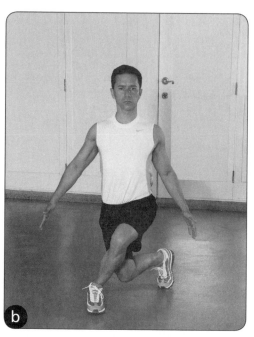

TRAINING TIP

Besides getting a great stretch, you will have to concentrate on waking up your nervous system to focus on balance. Stretch slowly on the way down into your lunge.

PLANKS WITH SHOULDER ABDUCTION

EXERCISE NOTES

- Complete the dynamic warm-up exercises before performing all three weight workouts in the Core Power Workout.
- Complete this exercise directly after performing curtsy lunges.

Start

Step 1: *(a)* Lie down on a mat in plank position with your forearms parallel to each other and your shoulders directly above your elbows.

Step 2: Keep your feet no more than hip-width apart.

Midpoint

Step 3: *(b)* Quickly use the muscles behind your left shoulder to rotate and abduct your arm up at the same right angle that it has while on the ground. When finished you should be looking down at the floor, still have your entire body in a plank, but have your left arm rotated out by your side at a right angle.

Finish

Step 4: Slowly lower your left arm back down to the floor and place it in its starting position on your forearm.

Step 5: Repeat on your right side and continue alternating reps.

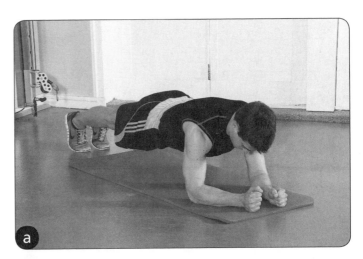

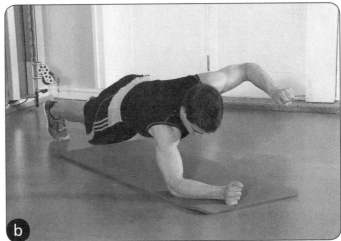

TRAINING TIP

This core challenge really fires up your obliques and postural muscles! Concentrate on keeping your balance and not letting your hips drop down toward the floor as you rotate.

BARBELL PUSH PRESSES

EXERCISE NOTES

- Complete the dynamic warm-up exercises first.
- This is the first exercise in the first workout of the Core Power Workout.

Start

Step 1: Hold on to a barbell just wider than shoulder-width apart.

Step 2: Place the barbell about 1 inch (2.5 cm) above your shoulders and collarbone.

Step 3: *(a)* Sit back into a quarter squat into your hips and heels while keeping the bar above your chest and shoulders.

Midpoint

Step 4: *(b)* Rapidly stand up straight, driving your feet into the floor and propelling the bar above your head into a shoulder press.

Finish

Step 5: Slowly decelerate the barbell back to the starting position as you move back into your quarter squat.

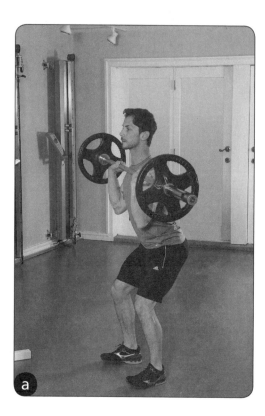 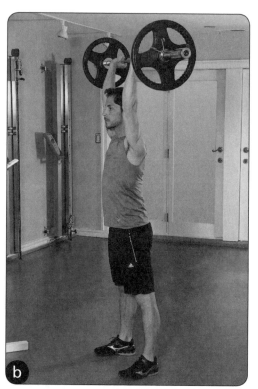

TRAINING TIP

The barbell push press is an excellent way to increase your core, leg, and shoulder strength and power all in one exercise! You can lift a heavier weight than you would typically be able to shoulder press, which makes it an effective way to increase muscle mass and strength.

BARBELL FRONT SQUATS

EXERCISE NOTES

- This is the second exercise in the Core Power Workout.
- Complete this exercise directly after performing barbell push presses.
- Because this is the second exercise in your superset, you will rest after completing it.

Start

Step 1: Stand with your feet hip-width apart and your knees slightly bent.

Step 2: *(a)* Step under the barbell and place it directly on your anterior deltoid and other shoulder muscles. The bar should touch the front of your neck right above your collarbone. (The bar is in the right position if you can balance it without touching it with your hands.)

Step 3: Grab the bar by folding your arms over it and holding it with your hands face down. Alternatively, you can use a traditional front squat grip by rotating your elbows forward, allowing your fingers and wrists to stretch back, and resting your palms on top of your shoulders while balancing the bar.

Midpoint

Step 4: Slowly breathe in, keep your chest and elbows lifted high, and sit back with your hips, keeping the weight on your heels.

Step 5: *(b)* Squat as deep as you can without rounding out your lower back, letting your heels come up, allowing your knees to go over your toes, dropping your chest, or going into a posterior pelvic tilt.

Finish

Step 6: Drive hard through your hips and heels to propel yourself back to the standing start position.

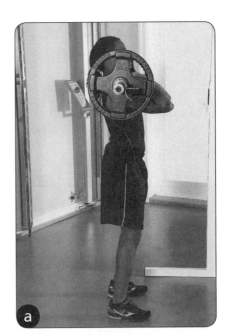

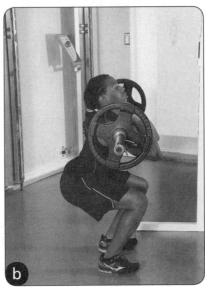

TRAINING TIP

Every serious weightlifter performs barbell back squats, but only the truly dedicated attempt front squats. This exercise forces you to train your body in a way that engages your core to the highest level. It also develops stronger quadriceps and promotes overall leg development. Start out lighter than you would a back squat and then work your way up after you master the form!

DUMBBELL ONE-LEG REACH TO ROWS

EXERCISE NOTES

- Complete the entire first superset three or four times before moving on to the second group of exercises.
- This is the first exercise in the second superset of the Core Power Workout.

Start

Step 1: Hold a dumbbell in your left hand and place your feet hip-width apart.

Step 2: *(a)* Sit back into your hips and begin to feel the stretch in your right hamstring and glutes as you lift your left leg off the ground and raise it straight back behind you.

Step 3: Allow your back (left) foot to point straight down as you extend your left arm with the dumbbell out in front of you pointed down diagonally to the floor.

Midpoint

Step 4: *(b)* Allow your upper body to bend forward to approximately a 45-degree angle while extending your left arm and left leg out straight.

Finish

Step 5: Pull the dumbbell back to your left oblique as you row the weight back to your hip using your back muscles. Stand back up to your starting position as you engage your right hamstring and glute muscles to pull yourself back up to the top.

Step 6: Repeat for the desired number of reps on your left side (trying not to touch your left foot to the floor) and then switch sides.

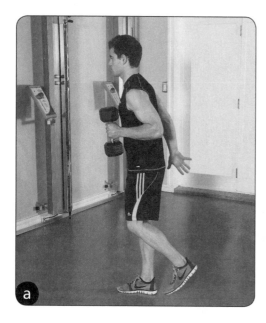 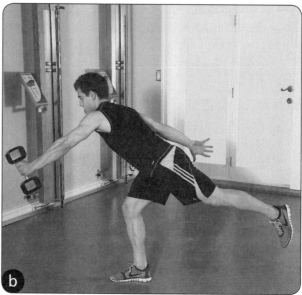

TRAINING TIP

This exercise challenges your core in both the sagittal plane and the transverse plane by forcing you to resist rotation and maintain your balance throughout the set. You also simultaneously work your upper and lower body in one movement!

BARBELL COMBAT TWISTS

EXERCISE NOTES

- This is the second exercise in the second superset of the first workout of the Core Power Workout.
- Complete this exercise directly after performing dumbbell one-leg reach to rows.
- Because this is the second exercise in your superset, you will rest after completing it.

Start

Step 1: Place a barbell in the corner on the floor where two walls intersect or into a device called a landmine.

Step 2: Hold the barbell up in the air at about a 45-degree angle or slightly higher from the ground. Grip it directly below where you place the weight plates with one hand below the other.

Step 3: Keep your knees slightly bent and your core engaged throughout the set.

Midpoint

Step 4: *(a)* Rotate the barbell to your left side by allowing your left elbow to bend into your body while keeping the right arm straight. Do not allow your body to rotate—resist the rotation!

Finish

Step 5: *(b)* Quickly swing the barbell in an arc to your right side by allowing your right elbow to bend into your right side and by keeping your left arm and elbow straight this time.

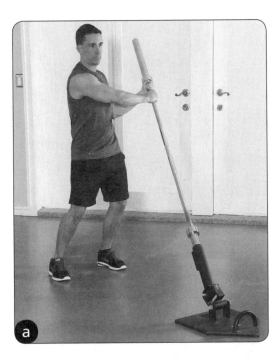
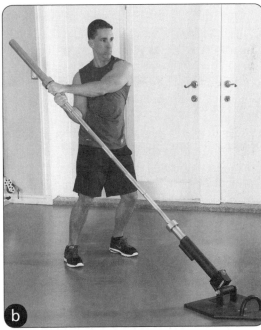

TRAINING TIP

This movement puts regular oblique twists and side crunches to shame! The biggest point to concentrate on here is not allowing your body to twist from side to side. You should look straight ahead throughout the set and allow only your arms to rotate.

CABLE KNEELING ROPE CHOPS

EXERCISE NOTES

- You should complete your entire Core Power Workout before moving on to this last exercise.
- This is the first and only exercise in this part of the Core Power Workout.
- After you complete this exercise, rest 60 to 90 seconds and repeat for two or three total sets.

Start

Step 1: Attach a rope to the lowest pulley attachment on a cable machine and stretch it out perpendicular from the machine so that it lies completely flat and outstretched.

Step 2: Place a padded mat on the floor directly in front of the outstretched rope.

Step 3: *(a)* Kneel on both knees on the mat and hold the rope with your left hand toward the top of the rope and your right hand close to the bottom of the rope. Both arms should be extended toward the cable machine.

Midpoint

Step 4: *(b)* Keep your glutes and core engaged throughout the set as you pull your left elbow across your left shoulder until your left hand moves directly in front of your left shoulder. Then quickly pull your left hand toward your left oblique and hip as you chop around and across with your right arm. Your right hand should end up directly in front of your left shoulder.

Finish

Step 5: After briefly pausing at the top, slowly decelerate the rope back down to its starting position without allowing your core to disengage or your body to rotate back toward the cable machine.

Step 6: Complete the desired number of reps and then turn around and face the opposite direction to repeat the movement on the other side.

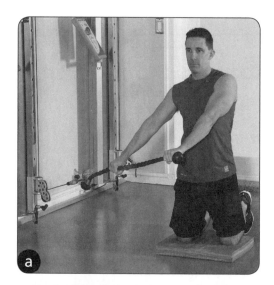

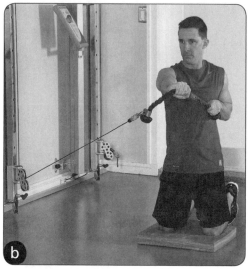

TRAINING TIP

This exercise is all about getting your first rep right. You may need to adjust your distance or the angle of your body until you find the best way to keep tension on the rope throughout the set without allowing your body to rotate back and forth. Remember, you're resisting the rotation, thereby working your obliques, lower back, and entire core in a safe, effective, and controlled manner.

T-TWIST PUSH-UPS

EXERCISE NOTES

- Complete the dynamic warm-up exercises first.
- This is the first exercise in the second workout of the Core Power Workout.

Start

Step 1: *(a)* Place both hands on the floor just past your shoulders and get up on the balls of your feet in a push-up position. Your feet should be about hip-width apart.

Step 2: *(b)* Decelerate your chest down toward the floor into a push-up without letting your hips sag.

Midpoint

Step 3: *(c)* As you push back up to the top, allow your entire body to rotate to the left so that your feet domino on to the outside of your left foot and the inside of your right foot. Your outside (right) arm should rise up above your shoulder to form a straight line with your left arm, which is supporting you on the bottom. Your entire body should form a T.

Finish

Step 4: After briefly pausing at the top, slowly decelerate the side of your body that is in the air down to the floor and back into a push-up position. Allow your feet to return to the balls of your feet as well.

Step 5: Complete another push-up but this time twist the other way. Continue alternating sides for the desired number of reps.

TRAINING TIP

Remember not to drop your hips as you open up to one side. Doing this will disengage your obliques and entire core, and you may lose balance. Take your time and work on becoming comfortable with the movement.

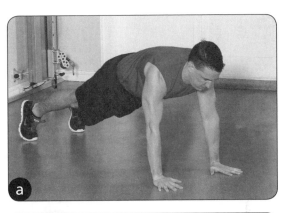

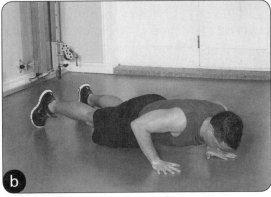

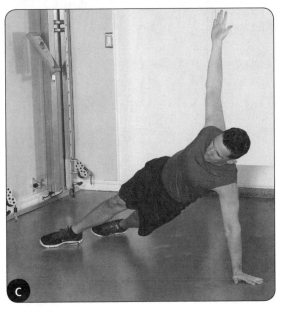

BARBELL ONE-LEG GOOD MORNINGS

EXERCISE NOTES

- This is the second exercise in the Core Power Workout.
- Complete this exercise directly after performing T-twist push-ups.

Start

Step 1: Stand with your feet hip-apart and place a slight bend in your knees.

Step 2: *(a)* Step under the barbell and place it directly on your trapezius muscles on your back below your neck. Hold the bar just wider than shoulder-width apart.

Midpoint

Step 3: *(b)* Slowly breathe in and sit back with your hips, keeping the weight on your heels as you lift your right leg off the ground and kick straight back with it.

Step 4: Stretch as deep you can into your left hip and hamstring while allowing your back to slowly lower toward the floor.

Finish

Step 5: Push through your hips and lift your upper body back up to standing position, squeezing the left glute area and not allowing the right foot to touch if possible (or just tap the ball of the right foot as you come to the top).

Step 6: Do all repetitions on one side before switching sides.

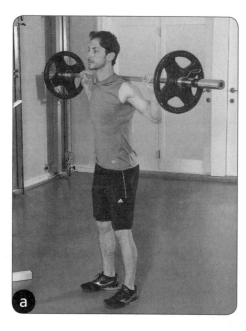 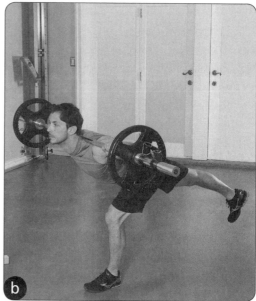

TRAINING TIP

The barbell one-leg good morning is a powerful exercise that you must take seriously. Concentrate on each rep and never stretch past the point of tension or round out your lower back at any point during the set. Maintain a flat back (neutral spine) and retract your shoulder blades for posture throughout the set. Also, make sure to keep your chest up and your core engaged.

STABILITY BALL ROLL-OUTS

EXERCISE NOTES

- This is the third exercise in the Core Power Workout.
- Complete this exercise directly after performing barbell one-leg good mornings.
- Because this is the third exercise in your tri-set, you will rest after completing it.

Start

Step 1: Place a cushioned mat under your knees as you kneel with both knees on the floor.

Step 2: *(a)* Place the ridge of both hands on a stability ball (or use an abs wheel) and press your palms together in front of you.

Step 3: Stretch out your body to a 45-degree angle with your arms and elbows straight in front of you.

Step 4: *(b)* Push the stability ball out in front of you by shifting your entire body forward until you feel your core engage tightly (stop before the point where your back arches). Your forearms should be firmly placed on the ball.

Midpoint

Step 5: Your body should be outstretched and stiff like a plank. At this point use your abs and core to pull your body back to the starting position without losing all the tension on your core.

Finish

Step 6: Pull back to the starting position and then slowly roll back out, repeating the same movement.

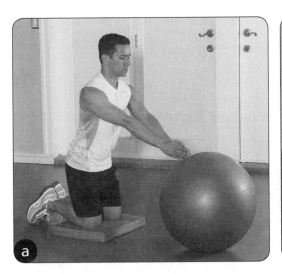
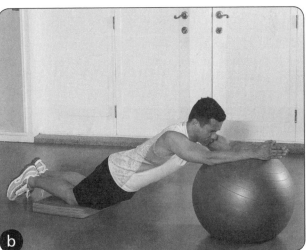

TRAINING TIP

This exercise can be done with a few variations. The easiest one is on both knees as described here. If that becomes too easy, you can use an abs wheel to roll out farther while maintaining the same form. Another way to make this exercise more challenging is to stand on the balls of your feet in a plank position while doing the roll-outs on a stability ball.

DUMBBELL ONE-ARM PRONE ROWS

EXERCISE NOTES

- Complete the entire first tri-set two or three times before moving on to the second group of exercises.
- This is the first exercise in second tri-set of the Core Power Workout.

Start

Step 1: Grab a dumbbell in your left hand and place your right hand on top of a bench.

Step 2: Walk both feet back until you are in a plank position with your shoulder and chest directly above your right hand.

Step 3: *(a)* Allow the weight in your left hand to stretch down directly below your left shoulder. Keep your core engaged and maintain a neutral spine so that you do not round out any part of your back.

Midpoint

Step 4: *(b)* Pull the dumbbell up to your left oblique using the muscles in your back behind your left shoulder. Do not let your biceps muscles take over the row.

Finish

Step 5: Slowly decelerate the weight back to the starting position while feeling your back and shoulder muscles stretch (without rounding your shoulders excessively). Keep your core engaged and your legs holding strong at hip- to shoulder-width apart.

Step 6: Repeat all reps on the left side before switching to the right.

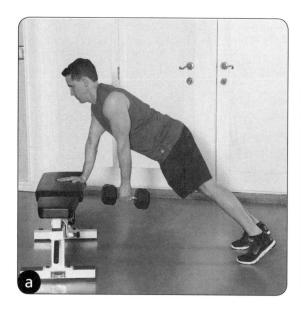
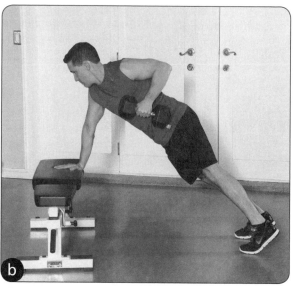

TRAINING TIP

The benefit of this great core exercise is that you really hit your obliques while simultaneously working your back postural muscles. Go slow and concentrate on each rep without letting your hips drop too low or rise up too high (maintain a strong plank position).

BARBELL OVERHEAD SQUATS

EXERCISE NOTES

- This is the second exercise in the second tri-set of the Core Power Workout.
- Complete this exercise directly after performing dumbbell one-arm prone rows.

Start

Step 1: *(a)* Grab a barbell with your hands wider than shoulder-width apart and raise it above your head.

Step 2: Stand with your feet shoulder-width apart and allow your hips to sit back slightly as you stand up straight.

Step 3: Let the barbell stretch open your chest and keep your elbows straight as the bar locks back into position above and behind your head. Pull your shoulder blades back for support. The barbell should not move from this position throughout the set.

Midpoint

Step 4: *(b)* Inhale and sit back into your hips into a squat, allowing the weight to fall back onto your heels.

Step 5: Continue to keep your chest up and look straight ahead with your chin parallel to the floor.

Finish

Step 6: Drive through your heels and hips to propel yourself back to your standing position.

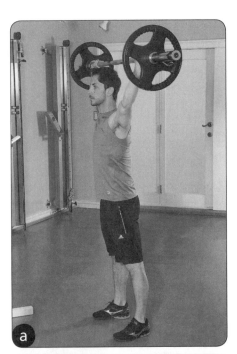

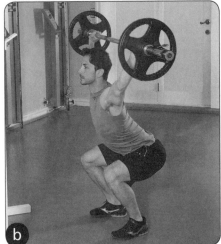

TRAINING TIP

This exercise is the real deal, and it will stretch you to your limits—literally. The biggest mistake that I see guys make during this exercise is letting their knees begin the movement by improperly shifting forward because they do not feel comfortable sitting back into their hips. To get more comfortable with the movement, put a box or bench behind you to learn to sit back into the squat. Just make sure that you do not let your body rest at the bottom or disengage your core. Start with an empty bar as a weight.

UNILATERAL BIRD DOGS

EXERCISE NOTES

- This is the third exercise in the second tri-set of the Core Power Workout.
- Complete this exercise directly after performing barbell overhead squats.
- Because this is the third exercise in your tri-set, you will rest after completing it.

Start

Step 1: Kneel down by placing both knees on a mat.

Step 2: Place your hands directly below your shoulders and point your fingers forward.

Step 3: *(a)* Look down toward the floor and maintain a neutral spine.

Step 4: Engage your core.

Midpoint

Step 5: *(b)* Simultaneously lift your right arm and right leg off the floor. Use your glutes and engage your shoulder to straighten both your right arm and your right leg so that they form a straight line down your body.

Finish

Step 6: Slowly breathe in and return your arm and leg to the starting position. (A more advanced way is to hold both your right knee and hand off the ground throughout the set.)

Step 7: Repeat all repetitions on your right side before switching to your left side.

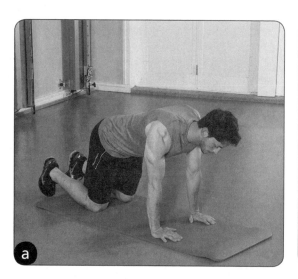
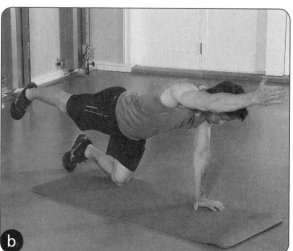

TRAINING TIP

This exercise is a lot harder than it looks. My big tip here is not to allow your body to cheat by leaning into the side that has your arm and knee placed on the floor. Stay level and work on tightening your core so that you don't tip over. Keep practicing and you'll get it!

CABLE LOW TO HIGH ROPE CHOPS

EXERCISE NOTES

- Complete the dynamic warm-up exercises first.
- This is the first exercise in the third workout of the Core Power Workout.
- This workout is circuit based, so you complete all five exercises in a row without resting.
- After you complete all five exercises you can rest for two or three minutes before repeating the entire circuit.

Start

Step 1: Attach a rope to a cable machine at the lowest pulley available.

Step 2: Grab the rope in both hands with your palms facing each other.

Step 3: *(a)* Step away from the cable machine so that tension is on the rope throughout the set.

Step 4: Tighten your core and step out in the transverse plane with the foot that is farther from the machine. Your foot should be perpendicular to the machine when it lands.

Midpoint

Step 5: *(b)* As your foot is landing in position out in front of you, use your core and both arms held out straight to chop the rope from a low position to about shoulder height. You should end the movement facing the foot that is turned out in front of you with an end of the rope in front of each shoulder. Your entire head and core should rotate to face away from the machine and toward the foot pointed out in front.

Finish

Step 6: Slowly return the rope to the starting position as both your front leg and core return to their original placement.

Step 7: Repeat all reps on one side before switching.

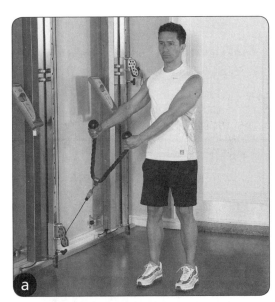

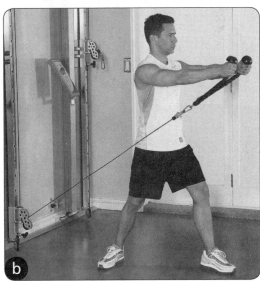

TRAINING TIP

This powerful core-based movement is fantastic in its application to sport. You need to be able to produce a lot of power from your initial movement to get your entire body moving as one, as well as to chop the rope up and across your body to shoulder height. Fight the urge to use just your arms to lift the rope. Your elbows should remain straight (but not locked) throughout the set.

MEDICINE BALL SLAMS

EXERCISE NOTES

- This is the second exercise in the circuit workout of the Core Power Workout.
- Complete this exercise directly after performing cable low to high rope chops.

Start

Step 1: Stand with your feet approximately shoulder-width apart and hold a medicine ball with both hands.

Step 2: *(a)* Raise the medicine ball overhead.

Midpoint

Step 3: *(b)* Quickly flex your core, sit back with your hips, and exhale while forcefully slamming the ball from overhead onto the mat between your feet by rapidly bringing both arms around and over your body. (Do not let go of the medicine ball at any time; hold on tight so that it doesn't bounce back up at you!)

Finish

Step 4: Stand back up to the starting position and raise the medicine ball back up overhead.

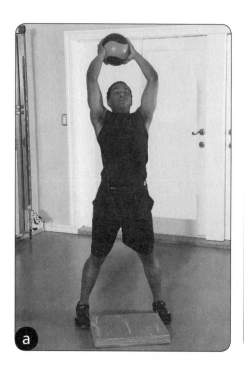
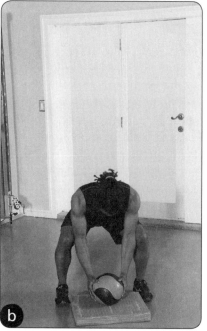

TRAINING TIP

Medicine ball slams are a great way to work your abs and core, almost as if you were performing a crunch. The difference is that this exercise is far more functional and is great for developing a lean, mean, and functionally fit midsection. Don't be afraid to slam the ball hard into the floor (use a mat if you're worried about the noise or impact on the floor).

SIDE PLANKS WITH REACH UNDER

EXERCISE NOTES

- This is the third exercise in the circuit workout of the Core Power Workout.
- Complete this exercise directly after performing medicine ball slams.

Start

Step 1: Lie on your right side and place your right elbow directly below your right shoulder. Your right forearm should lie on a mat perpendicular to your body.

Step 2: Stack your left foot on top of your right foot and place your top left arm straight up in the air so that it forms a line with the right arm below.

Step 3: *(a)* Now push your hips off the floor so that only your right forearm and right foot and ankle are in contact with the floor.

Midpoint

Step 4: *(b)* While maintaining your high hip position take the top (left) arm and reach under and around your body until you touch your right oblique and lower back area with your left palm.

Finish

Step 5: Bring your left arm back around your body and raise it back up straight in the air into its starting position.

Step 6: Repeat for the desired number of reps and then switch sides.

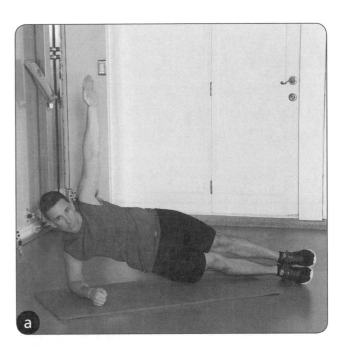

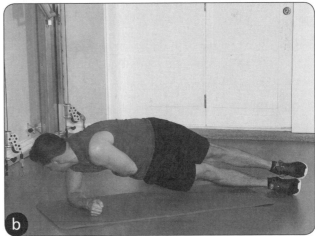

TRAINING TIP

The trick to completing this exercise properly is to make sure that your ear, shoulder, hip, knee, and ankle are all lined up perfectly straight when you are maintaining your static side plank position. This positioning will engage your body in its proper kinetic chain, allow you to complete the movement using the correct muscle groups, and strengthen your core to a greater degree.

DUMBBELL WALKING LUNGES WITH CHOP

EXERCISE NOTES

- This is the fourth exercise in the circuit workout of the Core Power Workout.
- Complete this exercise directly after performing side planks with reach under.

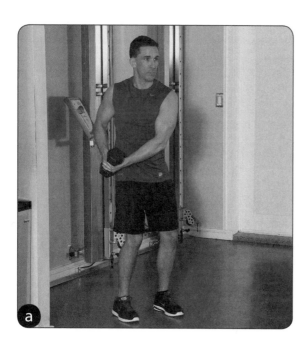
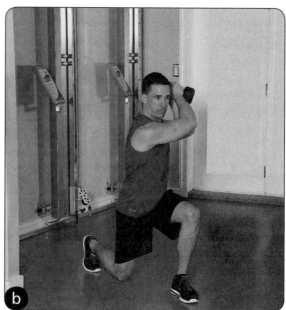

Start

Step 1: Standing with your feet hip-width apart, hold a single dumbbell with both hands gripping the handle (one hand may slightly overlap the other).

Step 2: *(a)* Place the dumbbell in front of your right hip.

Step 3: Lunge forward with your left leg by taking a large step forward with that leg and sitting into your left hip and heel.

Midpoint

Step 4: *(b)* As you sink deeply into your left hip while you're lunging, complete a reverse dumbbell chop by raising the dumbbell with both arms (slightly bent) directly above your left shoulder and away from your back (right) hip.

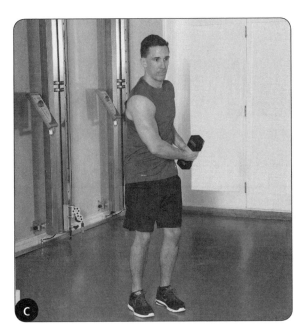

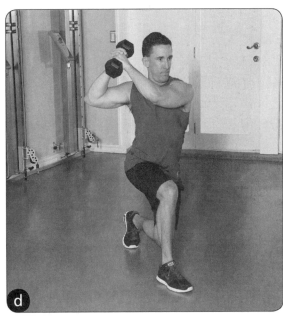

Finish

Step 5: *(c)* Step forward with your back (right) leg as your left hip and heel propel you up to a standing position, and return the dumbbell to your left hip. *(d)* Repeat this movement by lunging into your right leg and chopping the dumbbell over your right shoulder.

Step 6: Continue alternating sides until the set is complete.

TRAINING TIP

This exercise makes regular dumbbell walking lunges look like a walk in the park! The reverse dumbbell chop at the bottom of your lunge forces you to stay in the lunge longer, thus increasing the time under tension and improving both your core and leg strength. The added benefit of chopping the weight over the opposite shoulder of the back leg is that you will receive a greater stretch through the obliques and hip flexors of that side.

COBRAS

EXERCISE NOTES

- Complete this exercise after performing dumbbell walking lunges with chop.
- This is the fifth exercise in the circuit workout of the Core Power Workout.
- Because this is the final exercise of the circuit, you will rest two or three minutes after completing it before beginning the five-exercise circuit again.

Start

Step 1: Lie flat on your belly with your arms (palms down) outstretched overhead and your legs extended behind you.

Step 2: Look straight down at the floor throughout the set.

Step 3: *(a)* Lift your head, arms, and legs off the floor a few inches so that only your torso remains in contact with the floor.

Midpoint

Step 4: *(b)* Engage your glutes, lower back, and upper shoulders as you simultaneously raise both arms and legs off the floor as high as you can. As your arms reach their peak position, quickly pull your arms back beside your hips and point your thumbs up into the air (rotate your palms from facing the floor to facing away from your body).

Finish

Step 5: Slowly bring your arms back overhead and lower both arms and legs to the starting position above the floor.

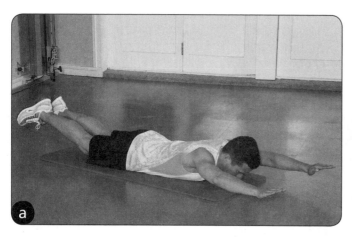
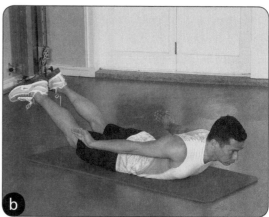

TRAINING TIP

This intense exercise strengthens many of the postural muscles that you can't see on your back side. Remember to engage your glutes and stretch open your chest (by squeezing your shoulder blades together) as you pull your arms and legs off the floor.

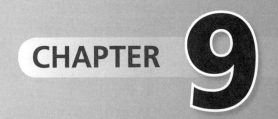

CHAPTER 9

Strength and Power Workout

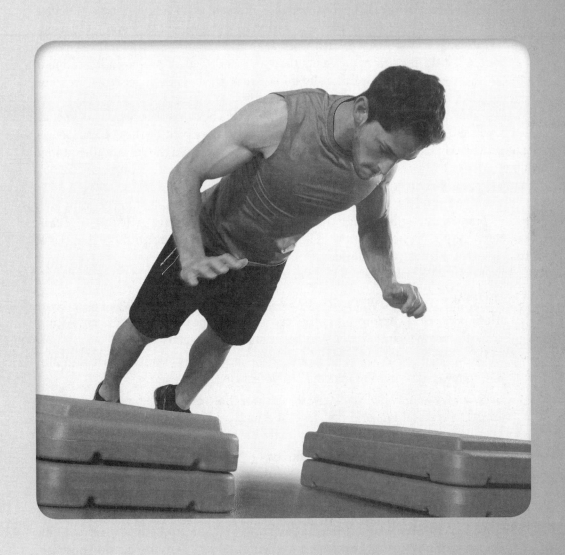

Being strong and being explosive are two different things. To me, being strong isn't too useful without having the athleticism to use that strength when it counts. For example, I've been practicing martial arts for over a decade and when it comes to a fight between two evenly skilled opponents, the guy who is strong and fast will typically take out an opponent who may be stronger but lacks explosive power.

You know explosive power when you see it.

You see it in the linebacker leveling a running back coming out of the backfield, a sumo wrestler toppling over his opponent with one lunge, or a Mike Tyson upper cut. Although you may not be using your newfound strength and power in competition, this workout will enable you to become a more fit and well-rounded athlete. You'll simply feel stronger, tighter, and faster.

You'll also know that you can move some serious weight without having to look like a Neanderthal in the gym. Basically, you'll be able to walk around having the quiet confidence of knowing that you can outlift most other guys you meet. And like I said, you won't sacrifice any quickness in the process.

You'll be able to do this because I'm going to have you add in some plyometrics and other fast-twitch muscle fiber movements that will push your body to new levels. This program is unlike any of the others in that you're most likely going to have to work your body in ways that it hasn't before.

Of course, adding new movements that your body hasn't prepared for is one of the best ways to develop new muscular and neurological strength, leading to a better overall physique and more functionally fit body.

If you haven't guessed yet, every program in this book has been created to challenge you in different ways to become better. It's not about picking the coolest-looking exercise but choosing the movements that are going to build the most well-rounded body possible. Make sure to use table 9.1 and tables 9.2 and 9.3 on page 152 as a basis to track your workouts.

I want your body to perform while you're hitting the weights, and I want your hard work to show right through the clothes that you're wearing. After all, why can't you have the best of both worlds? A strong, explosive physique with the muscles to match—that sounds good, doesn't it?

I thought so. Now let's check out the top tips and benefits of this program!

Top 10 Tips and Benefits of the Strength and Power Workout:

1. Be sure never to compromise proper form to lift a heavier weight. Form is king, and it's the one variable that can never change between sets.

2. Because this is a six-week program, make sure to ease into weeks 1 and 2 by doing fewer sets and not maxing out your lifts.

3. Although you may be familiar with many of these exercises, be sure to read the exercise descriptions and pay careful attention to the nuances and variations that differ from the typical movement pattern of the exercise.

4. Now that we have added some explosive plyometric movements, be sure to practice each move in a controlled manner. Although the concentric phase of plyometrics is meant to be done as quickly and explosively as possible, you want to keep your technique on point throughout the set.

5. If you ever think that your form is starting to falter, immediately discontinue any of your heavy or plyometric movements and return to the starting position.

6. Although you should be trying to increase your weight (or reps for body-weight exercises) lifted each week, don't be alarmed if you get stuck with a particular lift on a certain day and need to stay at the same weight for that week.

7. If an exercise doesn't feel right, go back and read the how-to description and look again at the details in the photos.

8. Remember that although you're not doing any typical abdominal exercises during this program, you are still working your core. Your abs and every other core muscle are being pushed to their limit with every heavy lift or plyometric move that you complete.

9. If a few months have passed since you've done any low-repetition strength work, then this is the program that you've been looking for. It will make you stronger and enable you to return to all your previous lifts and lift more weight with better form.

10. After the sixth week of consistent Strength and Power Workouts, you will find that you will feel not only stronger but also more athletic. You will feel as if you are ready to hit the NFL Combine!

Table 9.1 Strength and Power Workout, Workout Chart 1

Exercise	Sets	Reps	Tempo	Week 1	Week 2	Week 3	Week 4	Week 5	Week 6
W1. Skips in place	1	10	1-1-1-1	Weights					
W2. Speed skaters	1	20	1-0-1-0						
W3. Plank get-ups	1	10	1-1-1-1						
(Once warm-up exercises are completed, begin strength training.)									
1A. Plyometric box jumps	4	8-8-5-3	0						
1B. Plyometric box push-ups	4	10-8	0						
(Rest 2–3 minutes and repeat exercises 1A and 1B.)									
2A. Barbell inverted pronated rows	4	10-8	2-0-1-1						
2B. Barbell backward lunges	4	2 × 8	3-0-1-1						
(Rest 2–3 minutes and repeat exercises 2A and 2B.)									

Table 9.2 Strength and Power Workout, Workout Chart 2

Exercise	Sets	Reps	Tempo	Week 1	Week 2	Week 3	Week 4	Week 5	Week 6
W1. Skips in place	1	10	1-1-1-1			Weights			
W2. Speed skaters	1	20	1-0-1-0						
W3. Plank get-ups	1	10	1-1-1-1						
(Once warm-up exercises are completed, begin strength training.)									
1A. Dumbbell one-arm snatches	4	2 × 8-5	1-0-1-1						
1B. Alternate split lunge jumps	3-4	20-16	0						
(Rest 2–3 minutes and repeat exercises 1A and 1B.)									
2A. Cable supinated lat pull-downs	4	8-5	2-0-1-1						
2B. Barbell deadlifts from boxes	4	8-5-5-3	3-0-1-1						
(Rest 2–3 minutes and repeat exercises 2A and 2B.)									

Table 9.3 Strength and Power Workout, Workout Chart 3

Exercise	Sets	Reps	Tempo	Week 1	Week 2	Week 3	Week 4	Week 5	Week 6
W1. Skips in place	1	10	1-1-1-1			Weights			
W2. Speed skaters	1	20	1-0-1-0						
W3. Plank get-ups	1	10	1-1-1-1						
(Once warm-up exercises are completed, begin strength training.)									
1A. Dumbbell floor chest presses	5	5	3-0-1-1						
1B. Barbell deep box squats	5	5	3-0-1-1						
(Rest 2–3 minutes and repeat exercises 1A and 1B.)									
2A. Cable pronated wide-grip seated rows	4	8-5	2-0-1-1						
2B. Cable rope pull-throughs	4	8	2-0-1-1						
2C. Cable alternating horizontal chops	3	20	0						
(Rest 2–3 minutes and repeat exercises 2A, 2B, and 2C.)									

SKIPS IN PLACE

EXERCISE NOTES

Complete the dynamic warm-up exercises before performing all three weight workouts in the Strength and Power Workout.

Start

Step 1: Stand with your feet hip-width apart and your arms by your sides.

Step 2: *(a)* Raise your right knee up in the air to about hip height while simultaneously raising your left arm at about a right angle until your hand goes at, or slightly above, your head.

Midpoint

Step 3: *(b)* Bring your right knee and left arm down as you quickly raise up the opposite limbs, taking your left knee to hip height (or higher) and your right arm up in the air.

Finish

Step 4: After you get the movement pattern down you can speed up the motion and turn it into skips during which you leave the ground with each repetition.

Step 5: Repeat for 20 seconds.

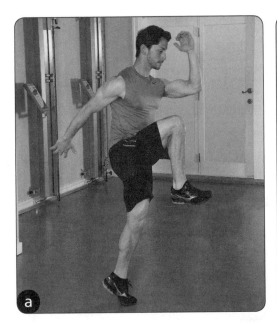
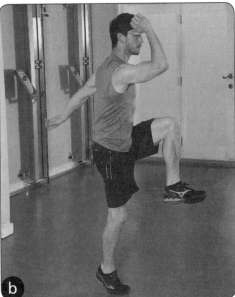

TRAINING TIP

Although most people think that they'll look silly doing this exercise, it is one of the top neurological warm-ups that almost every professional athlete does before a competition. Practice at home before you hit the gym if you think that your coordination may need a few practice runs.

SPEED SKATERS

EXERCISE NOTES

- Complete the dynamic warm-up exercises before performing all three weight workouts in the Strength and Power Workout.
- Complete this exercise directly after performing skips in place.

Start

Step 1: Stand with your feet hip-width apart and hold your arms up in front of your chest.

Step 2: *(a)* Quickly leap to your right side and land on your right foot while maintaining balance (do not allow your left foot to touch).

Midpoint

Step 3: *(b)* Sit back into your right hip and then propel yourself off the right foot, jumping parallel or laterally over onto your left foot.

Finish

Step 4: Sit back into your left hip and jump back to your right side. Repeat back and forth for 20 repetitions.

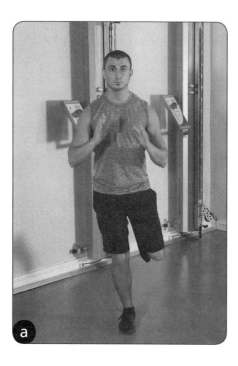
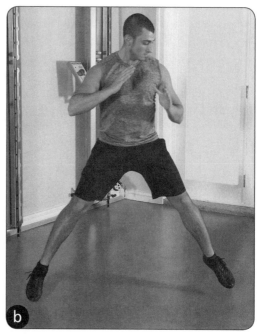

TRAINING TIP

This exercise works on balance and lateral knee stability. It's an excellent move that will strengthen and stabilize your leg joints while priming you for your workout. Make sure that you are balanced at all times and do not make your next leap to the opposite side until you gain complete control.

PLANK GET-UPS

EXERCISE NOTES

- Complete the dynamic warm-up exercises before performing all three weight workouts in the Strength and Power Workout.
- Complete this exercise directly after performing speed skaters.

Start

Step 1: *(a)* Lie on a mat in a plank position with your forearms parallel to each other and your shoulders directly above your elbows.

Step 2: Keep your feet no more than hip-width apart.

Midpoint

Step 3: *(b)* After you feel as if you have engaged your core, draw your right arm off the mat and place your palm down directly under your right shoulder (where your right elbow just was).

Step 4: *(c)* Next, pull your left arm off the mat and place that hand directly under your left shoulder as you prop yourself up into a push-up plank position.

Finish

Step 5: Lower your right arm back down to the floor by placing your right forearm back into the starting position. Repeat that movement with your left arm.

Step 6: Repeat by now lifting your left arm off the floor and then your right to prop yourself back up again into a push-up plank position. On the way back down lower your left arm first and then place your right arm back into the starting position. Alternate which arm starts each time.

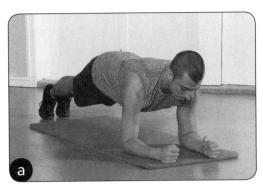

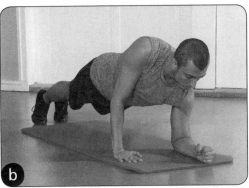

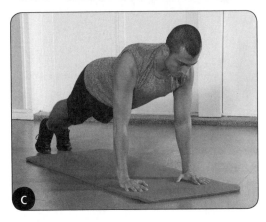

TRAINING TIP

I like this exercise because it challenges your entire upper body, including your core. It also fires up your nervous system to get you ready for your big Strength and Power Workouts! Don't be too concerned if you mess up on which arm comes up first. Just do the opposite arm the next time and keep going!

PLYOMETRIC BOX JUMPS

EXERCISE NOTES

- Complete the dynamic warm-up exercises first.
- This is the first exercise in the first workout of the Strength and Power Workout.

Start

Step 1: Place a box in front of you at a height that you feel comfortable jumping up onto.

Step 2: Stand with your feet hip-width apart and no more than 1 foot (30 cm) away from the box.

Step 3: *(a)* Sit back into your hips into a quarter squat, pulling your arms back by your sides.

Midpoint

Step 4: *(b)* Explode off the balls of your feet and throw your arms up as you leap off the ground up onto the box.

Finish

Step 5: *(c)* Absorb the impact down onto the box by doing a partial squat.

Step 6: Step down (do not jump backward) off the box and then set up for your next jump. You can try to increase the height of the box with each set.

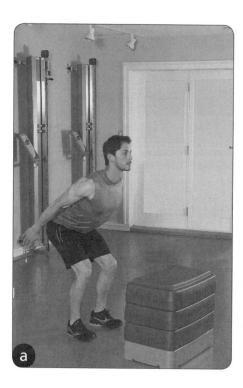 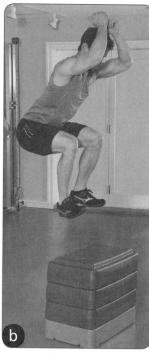 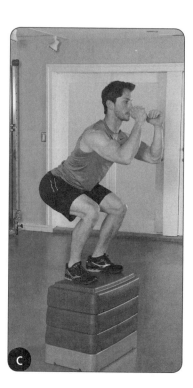

TRAINING TIP

This excellent plyometric exercise will help you maximize your fast-twitch muscle fiber recruitment and work on your explosiveness. My tip here is to concentrate on jumping off both feet at the same time to get the most out of your jump.

PLYOMETRIC BOX PUSH-UPS

EXERCISE NOTES

- This is the second exercise in the Strength and Power Workout.
- Complete this exercise directly after performing plyometric box jumps.
- Because this is the second exercise in the superset, you will rest before repeating.

Start

Step 1: Place two boxes (you can use stacked weight plates instead) on the ground with about 1 foot (30 cm) of space between them.

Step 2: Get into a push-up position with one hand on each box so that your upper body is slightly inclined.

Step 3: *(a)* Maintain a flat back (neutral spine) and decelerate down into a push-up on the boxes.

Step 4: *(b)* When you push back up to the top, accelerate so that you literally propel yourself up in the air and your hands leave the boxes.

Midpoint

Step 5: *(c)* When you bring your hands back down allow them to land inside the two boxes, absorbing your impact and immediately dropping back down into your next push up.

Step 6: Quickly push up as fast as you can and again propel yourself off the floor and up onto the boxes for your next push-up.

Finish

Step 7: Immediately decelerate down into the next push-up to repeat the process.

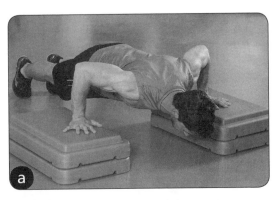

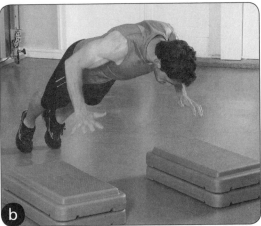

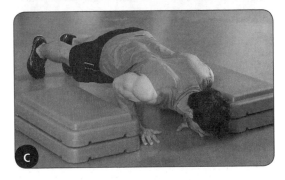

TRAINING TIP

And you thought some of the other chest exercises were tough! This exercise allows you to start at any height you want and lets you move up as you get more comfortable. The higher the boxes are, the greater the force and deceleration you'll need. Try to flow from one push-up to the next without stopping at either the bottom or the top position. This flow will allow your natural stretch–reflex response to kick in and help propel you up into the air with each rep!

BARBELL INVERTED PRONATED ROWS

EXERCISE NOTES

- Complete the entire first superset three or four times before moving on to the second group of exercises.
- This is the first exercise in the second superset of the Strength and Power Workout.

Start

Step 1: Set up a Smith machine or barbell bench press station so that the barbell is in a fixed and secure position.

Step 2: After you have placed the bar where you want it (the higher the bar is, the easier the exercise will be to complete), slide under the bar facing up to the ceiling.

Step 3: *(a)* Grip the bar slightly wider than shoulder-width apart and stretch your body out under the bar so that your chest lines up directly under it. Make sure that your knees are straight and that your toes point up to the ceiling.

Midpoint

Step 4: *(b)* With your hips lifted and your core and glutes engaged throughout the set, pull your chest up to the bar by squeezing your back muscles and pulling your shoulder blades together.

Finish

Step 5: Allow your body to lower slowly toward the floor without touching, continue to keep tension on your back, and do not allow your shoulders to round forward.

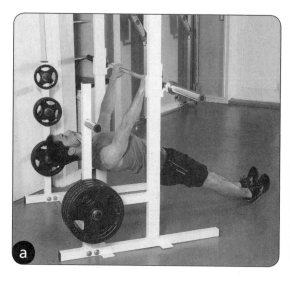 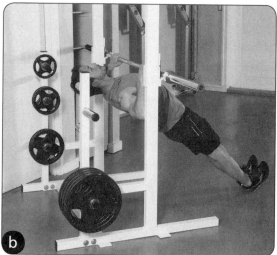

TRAINING TIP

The main point here is that you keep your entire body stiff in an upside-down plank position with your core and glutes engaged so that your back muscles can do their job of pulling your chest up to the bar. Also, focus more on squeezing your shoulder blades together and less on using your arms to pull your chest up to the bar.

BARBELL BACKWARD LUNGES

EXERCISE NOTES

- This is the second exercise in the second superset of the first workout of the Strength and Power Workout.
- Complete this exercise directly after performing barbell inverted pronated rows.
- Because this is the second exercise in your superset, you will rest after completing it.

Start

Step 1: Stand with your feet shoulder-width apart and your knees slightly bent.

Step 2: *(a)* Step under the barbell and place it directly on your trapezius muscles below your neck. Hold the bar just beyond shoulder-width apart.

Step 3: Maintain a flat back (neutral spine) and retract your shoulder blades for posture throughout the set. Also, make sure to keep your chest up and your chin parallel to the floor.

Midpoint

Step 4: Slowly breathe in and sit back with your hips, keeping the weight on your front heel as you step back with your left foot. Land on just the ball of your foot (the heel of the back foot should never touch the floor).

Step 5: *(b)* Sit into your right hip and heel and decelerate your left knee down until it almost touches the floor.

Finish

Step 6: Push as hard you can through your right hip and heel as you step your left foot back to its starting position.

Step 7: Repeat on the same side for the desired number of reps and then switch.

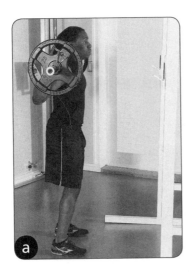 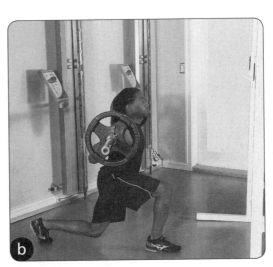

TRAINING TIP

The biggest mistakes that I see guys make during this exercise are failing to step back far enough (your legs should look like right angles at the bottom of your lunge), placing too much weight on the back foot and allowing the heel to touch, and not sitting back enough into the front hip. If you can concentrate on correcting those points you will get the most benefit out of this great leg exercise!

DUMBBELL ONE-ARM SNATCHES

EXERCISE NOTES

- Complete the dynamic warm-up exercises first.
- This is the first exercise in the second workout of the Strength and Power Workout.

Start

Step 1: Stand with your feet about shoulder-width apart and hold a single dumbbell in your right hand between your legs.

Step 2: *(a)* Allow your knees to bend slightly and sit back with your hips so that you can feel your hamstrings and glutes stretch. Let your right arm hang straight with the weight between your legs.

Midpoint

Step 3: *(b)* As you push forward and up with your hips into a standing position, pull the dumbbell up toward your right shoulder as if you are doing a one-arm upright row with your right palm facing your chest and shoulder on that side. At this point you should be moving so explosively that your heels are leaving the floor and you feel as if you are jumping up.

Step 4: *(c)* Without stopping the motion, snap the dumbbell up over your right shoulder by flipping your right palm to face forward and allowing the momentum of your pull to keep going straight overhead.

Finish

Step 5: Briefly pause at the top without letting the dumbbell twist and then slowly decelerate the dumbbell back down to your shoulder and then between your legs for the next rep on your right side.

Step 6: Finish all the repetitions on your right side and then switch.

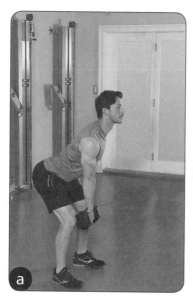 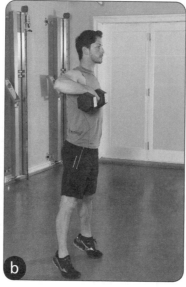 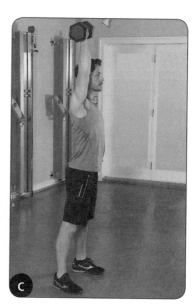

TRAINING TIP

Remember that this is not an upright row to a shoulder press, although that's what it may look like if you slow down the motion. You are exploding up with your hips and pulling the weight so fast that it just pops over your shoulder and above your head without your having to press it. With a little practice and focus, you'll master this explosive movement in no time!

BARBELL DEADLIFTS FROM BOXES

EXERCISE NOTES

- This is the second exercise in the second superset of the second workout of the Strength and Power Workout.
- Complete this exercise directly after performing cable supinated lat pull-downs.
- Because this is the second exercise in the superset, you will rest before repeating.

Start

Step 1: Set up two 4- to 6-inch (10 to 15 cm) boxes under a barbell so that the weight plates on the barbell rest on the middle of them.

Step 2: Stand over the barbell with your feet shoulder-width apart.

Step 3: Grip the barbell slightly wider apart than your knees and have one hand facing away from you and the other facing toward you (alternate grip).

Step 4: *(a)* Keeping your core engaged sit back with your hips into a squat while maintaining good posture (keep your chest up) and keeping your weight on your heels. Your back or hips should not round out. If they do, add an additional box to increase the height.

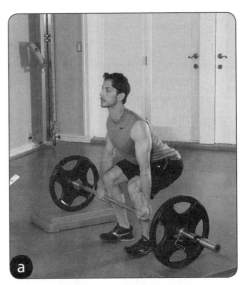

Midpoint

Step 5: *(b)* Look straight ahead throughout the set and make sure that the bar is in tight to your shins as you drive through your heels and pull the bar up to your quads. At the top keep your shoulders pulled back and squeeze your glutes together.

Finish

Step 6: Slowly sit back with your hips, keep the weight on your heels, and keep your back neutral as you lower the bar down to the bottom.

Step 7: Set the barbell down on the boxes and then get yourself ready for your next repetition.

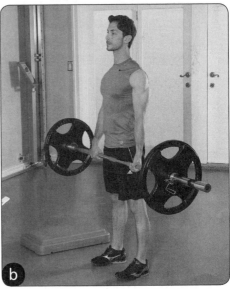

TRAINING TIP

The reason that I have you pulling from boxes is that I see too many guys using improper form and rounding out their backs at the bottom of this movement because of poor flexibility. By propping up the bar just 4 to 6 inches (10 to 15 cm), we can decrease the chance for injury while still getting a lot out of this excellent strength-based movement. When you think that your flexibility has improved, meaning that you can sit into a deep squat without your heels coming up or your hips tilting backward into a posterior pelvic tilt, you can lower the barbell down a level.

DUMBBELL FLOOR CHEST PRESSES

EXERCISE NOTES

- Complete the dynamic warm-up exercises first.
- This is the first exercise in the third workout of the Strength and Power Workout.

Start

Step 1: Sit on a mat on the floor holding two dumbbells on the top of your thighs.

Step 2: Lie backward and kick the dumbbells back until they rest on your chest.

Step 3: Keep your feet pulled into your hips so that the soles of your feet rest on the floor as if you are getting ready to do a sit-up.

Step 4: *(a)* Rotate your palms away from you so that the heads of the dumbbells are directly above your chest and shoulders. Your entire triceps area should be in contact with the ground so that your arms are just resting in place at right angles.

Midpoint

Step 5: *(b)* Squeeze your pectoral muscles and press the weights directly over your chest. Allow the dumbbells to come together in an arc, but do not bang them against each other at the top.

Finish

Step 6: Slowly decelerate the weights back to the starting position while feeling your chest and shoulder muscles stretch. Keep the tension on your chest the whole time and maintain stability in your shoulder joints. The difference with this exercise on the floor is that you will allow your arms to rest on the floor at right angles between reps for three or four seconds before you press back up again.

Step 7: Continuing pressing and resting after each repetition.

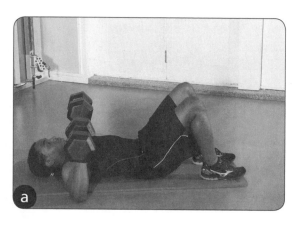 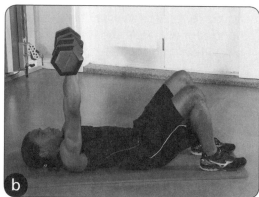

TRAINING TIP

The point of this exercise is to work from a pure strength standpoint. By allowing your arms to rest down on the floor between reps, you are eliminating the stretch–reflex response, which typically helps you to spring the weight back up for your next push. By taking out the rebound, you are forcing your pectorals as well as your other upper-body pushing muscles to work harder.

BARBELL DEEP BOX SQUATS

EXERCISE NOTES

- This is the second exercise of the Strength and Power Workout.
- Complete this exercise directly after performing dumbbell floor chest presses.
- Because this is the second exercise in the superset, you will rest before repeating.

Start

Step 1: Stand with your feet shoulder-width apart, your knees slightly bent, and your heels about 3 inches (8 cm) away from a box that you set up behind you. (The box should be about 12 inches [30 cm] high or less so that you can squat much deeper than parallel.)

Step 2: *(a)* Step under the barbell and place it directly on your trapezius muscles below your neck. Hold the bar just beyond shoulder-width apart.

Midpoint

Step 3: Slowly breathe in and sit back with your hips, keeping the weight on your heels. Maintain a flat back (neutral spine) and retract your shoulder blades for posture throughout the set. Also, make sure to keep your chest up and your chin parallel to the floor.

Step 4: *(b)* Squat down until you sit on the box but do not disengage your core or relax your body. If you begin rounding out your lower back, letting your heels come up, dropping your chest, or going into a posterior pelvic tilt, then the box is too low or you have too much weight on the bar. (First, take off some weight and try again. If you still make any of those mistakes, increase the height of the box.)

Finish

Step 5: Push as hard you can through your hips and heels, exploding back up to the standing start position.

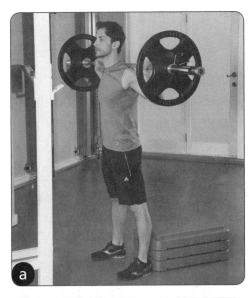

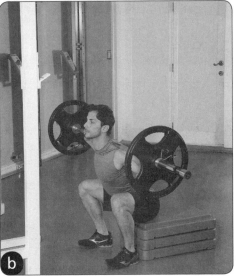

TRAINING TIP

Deep squats will enable you to increase strength in the most vulnerable and weakest position of your squat when you are parallel or below. By squatting deeper than parallel, you must go lighter in weight, but you will engage more muscle fiber to a greater degree and you can work on your explosiveness at the bottom of the movement as you drive back up to the top.

CABLE PRONATED WIDE-GRIP SEATED ROWS

EXERCISE NOTES

- Complete the entire first superset three or four times before moving on to the second group of exercises.
- This is the first exercise in the second tri-set of the Strength and Power Workout.

Start

Step 1: Affix a straight lat bar attachment to a seated row machine and grip it wider than shoulder-width apart using an overhand pronated grip while seated on the bench.

Step 2: With your knees bent place both feet against the footrest of the machine, engage your core, and retract your shoulder blades.

Step 3: *(a)* Push back with both legs to your starting position while maintaining a neutral spine and good posture. Ensure that you have a small bend in your knees throughout the set.

Midpoint

Step 4: *(b)* Concentrate on squeezing your shoulder blades back and stretching open your chest as you complete your first repetition by pulling the bar into your chest.

Finish

Step 5: Without allowing your shoulder blades or back to round forward, return your arms to their extended starting position. Maintain tension on your back muscles at all times.

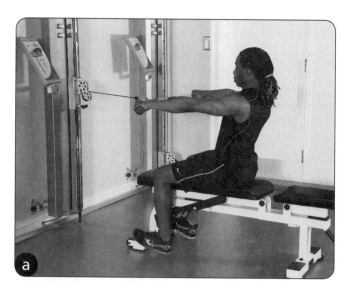

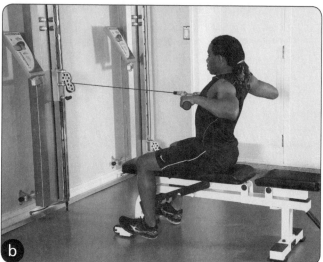

TRAINING TIP

Although you cannot lift quite as much weight using an overhand wide grip and pulling it into your chest, this exercise is the perfect complement to your heavy floor chest presses. It will balance out the muscles in your upper body and help correct postural deviations if you have rounded shoulders or a weak upper back compared with your chest. Make sure that you don't round your back as you return the weight toward the weight stack, and you'll be fine.

CABLE ROPE PULL-THROUGHS

EXERCISE NOTES

- This is the second exercise in the second tri-set of the third workout of the Strength and Power Workout.
- Complete this exercise directly after performing cable pronated wide-grip seated rows.

Start

Step 1: Attach a rope to the bottom pulley of a cable tower.

Step 2: Stand over the rope facing away from the machine and then grip both sides just below the ends as you step out about 2 feet (60 cm) from the pulley (keep your arms straight throughout the set).

Step 3: Keeping a flat back (neutral spine), retract your shoulder blades and place a slight bend in your knees.

Midpoint

Step 4: (a) Keep the weight on your heels and allow your hips to stretch backward (with up to a 20-degree bend in your knees) until you can't stretch your hamstrings and glutes anymore. Your upper body will lower a little, but the hips always move first and dictate how low you go. You will also feel the rope and your arms stretch through your legs toward the pulley.

Finish

Step 5: (b) Squeeze your glutes, push your hips forward, and pull your upper body back to the starting position before starting the next repetition. Exhale as you exert force and lift up. Remember not to pull with your arms or bend your elbows to pull back into the starting position.

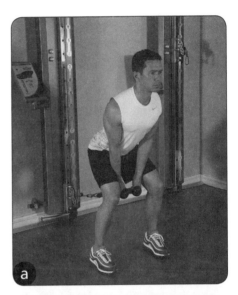

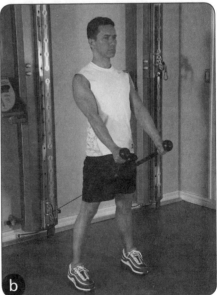

TRAINING TIP

If you recognize that you may not master this movement the first time you try it, you'll be way ahead of the game. The key points are to feel your hips stretch backward as you lower and then to swing your hips forward (as in a kettlebell swing) as you squeeze your glutes and stand up tall. Also, keep your arms straight with a tight grip throughout the set; they don't move because the focus is on your lower body and hips.

CABLE ALTERNATING HORIZONTAL CHOPS

EXERCISE NOTES

- This is the third exercise in the second tri-set of the third workout of the Strength and Power Workout.
- Complete this exercise directly after performing cable rope pull-throughs (three sets only).
- Because this is the last exercise in your tri-set, you will rest after completing it.

Start

Step 1: Attach a single handle on a cable tower at shoulder height.

Step 2: Grab the handle in both hands and interlock your fingers or wrap one hand over the other.

Step 3: Facing the cable pulley, step back about 3 feet (90 cm) so that you have plenty of room to chop to each side. Keep a slight bend in your knees throughout the set and engage your core. Look straight ahead and keep your elbows straight but not locked out throughout the set.

Midpoint

Step 4: *(a)* Without rotating your hips, chop your arms powerfully across your chest to your left side until the cable stretches across your right shoulder. Exhale forcefully as you chop.

Step 5: *(b)* Without pausing, quickly chop across your body to your right side until the cable stretches across your left shoulder.

Finish

Step 6: Maintain your posture and continue repeating from side to side for the desired number of reps.

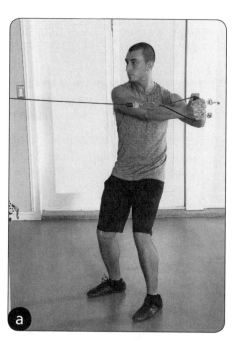

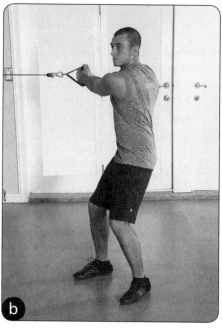

TRAINING TIP

You're going to have to resist the urge to move your feet and hips as you're forcefully chopping to each side. Also, remember not to let the weight move you. You are in control, so the cable should not slingshot you back to the middle after each chop. Lastly, do not stop in the middle after each repetition; instead, let each rep flow into the next to maintain momentum.

CHAPTER 10

Hard Gainer's Workout

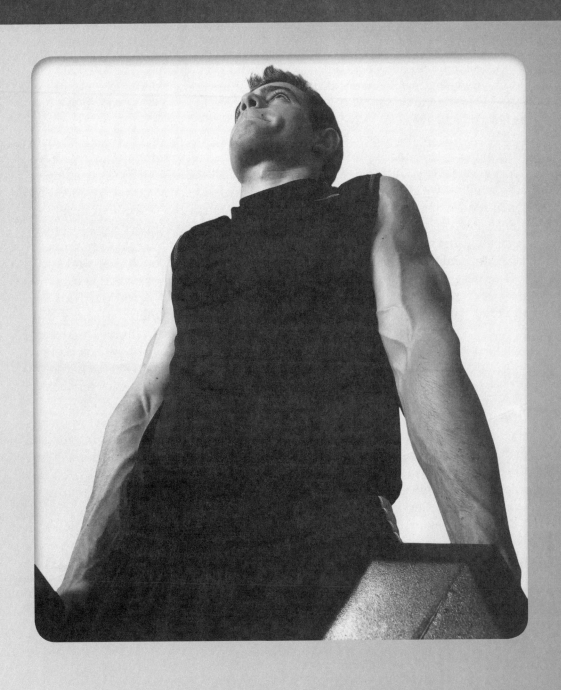

understand how frustrating it can be to have a difficult time packing on muscle. You can't understand how you're putting in your time at the gym and not getting the results that you believe you deserve to see. Although it may not be easy for you to put on lean muscle or bulk up, there is an answer that will allow you to break free of your genetic hardship.

The solution to your problem lies in your nutrition and exercise program design.

In terms of nutrition you must consume more calories that your body expends per day. Although this seems rather simplistic, it's nonetheless the truth. The best way to do this is to keep a food journal just as you would to lose weight, but in this case the goal is to pack it on.

I recommend breaking up your meals so that they are evenly spaced over the course of the day. That way you can add another 100 calories per meal and still have time to digest the calories between feedings. The key to all these nutritional aspects is consistency. Many guys believe that they are eating a ton of food, but for the most part they are overeating at a few big meals and then being inconsistent and not timing their intake the rest of the time.

If you still aren't gaining weight after a full week of adding 100 calories per meal, add another 100 calories per meal for the second week. The alternative is adding another meal if you are already taking in too many calories at each sitting. The easiest way to boost calories is by adding more healthy fat to your diet, such as olive oil and avocado.

Also, at this point in the game don't worry about putting on fat. If you're a true hard gainer you'll find it difficult to put on muscle, never mind doing it without adding any fat to your frame. The best plan of attack for anyone trying to add size is to gain the weight first (muscle and a little fat). Then, when you've added as much muscle as you'd like, you can begin to trim away the fat without dropping your calories too low or decreasing your heavy lifting days. I have used this plan personally and implemented it in many of my clients' programs. Make sure to use table 10.1 and tables 10.2 and 10.3 on page 172 as a basis to track your workouts.

The next aspect that we need to look at is the design of your exercise program. Real hard gainers should never work out two days in a row. A rest day between workouts will allow them to recover from their previous workout, regenerate, and rebuild bigger muscles. Therefore, in this program I developed a three-day-a-week weight-training program that will target every muscle in your body. You will be using specific and straightforward compound movements that will enable you to lift heavy amounts of weight for the proper sets and repetitions to pack on muscle scientifically.

You may even have to resist the urge to work out more when you see yourself starting to pack on muscle, but remember that the rest days allow you to grow. It may seem counterintuitive that to get bigger and bulk up you must be in the gym fewer days per week, but it's the truth for a hard gainer looking to add size and thickness to his physique. After you accept this fact, you will be well on your way to bigger and better muscle gains.

Now that you know what's in store for you during this six-week Hard Gainer's Workout, I'll leave you with a few tips, tricks, and benefits that will permit you to maximize every fragment of muscle-building potential that you have in your body.

Top 10 Tips and Benefits of the Hard Gainer's Workout:

1. Remember, for hard gainers rest is just as important as the workout itself.

2. Aim for eight to nine hours of sleep per night to maximize growth.

3. Add additional calories to each meal to fuel muscle growth.

4. Drink a carbohydrate and protein shake (4:1 ratio) before and after your workout so that you are never at a deficit and can immediately begin rebuilding your body.

5. Stay consistent with your eating. Unlike with your training days in the gym, you can never take a day off from eating the amount and quality of calories that you should be consuming. Track your daily eating and your weekly progress.

6. Aim to increase the amount of weight that you lift each week (without compromising form, of course).

7. Although you want to keep your rest time consistent, you can give yourself an extra minute of rest if you think that your heart rate is still too high for you to recover enough to complete your next set at your maximum capacity.

8. Don't listen to anyone who tells you that you need to be training every day of the week to pack on size. Although that type of routine may work for some people, if you're truly a hard gainer it will only hurt your progress.

9. Make every workout count. As they say, "Go hard, go heavy, or go home." Although I don't want you ever to use improper form or push yourself past a level that isn't safe, I want you to understand the importance of overloading your current capacity to stimulate new growth.

10. By the end of the Hard Gainer's Workout routine you should find that your T-shirts and jeans are fitting snugger than they did just six weeks ago!

Table 10.1 Hard Gainer's Workout, Workout Chart 1

Exercise	Sets	Reps	Tempo	Week 1	Week 2	Week 3	Week 4	Week 5	Week 6
W1. Spidermans	1	20	1-0-1-1	Weights					
W2. One-leg dynamic bridging	1	2 × 12	2-0-1-1						
W3. Plank one-arm reach-outs	1	20	1-1-1-1						
(Once warm-up exercises are completed, begin strength training.)									
1A. Barbell incline chest presses	4	8-5	3-0-1-1						
1B. Barbell Romanian deadlifts	4	8-5	3-0-1-1						
(Rest 2–3 minutes and repeat exercises 1A and 1B.)									
2A. Barbell bent-over rows	4	8-5	2-0-1-1						
2B. Barbell front squats	4	8-5	3-0-1-1						
(Rest 2–3 minutes and repeat exercises 2A and 2B.)									

Table 10.2 Hard Gainer's Workout, Workout Chart 2

Exercise	Sets	Reps	Tempo	Week 1	Week 2	Week 3	Week 4	Week 5	Week 6
W1. Spidermans	1	20	1-0-1-1	Weights					
W2. One-leg dynamic bridging	1	2 × 12	2-0-1-1						
W3. Plank one-arm reach-outs	1	20	1-1-1-1						
(Once warm-up exercises are completed, begin strength training.)									
1A. Barbell military shoulder presses	3	10	3-0-1-0						
1B. Barbell box step-ups	3	2 × 10-8	1-0-1-0						
(Rest 2–3 minutes and repeat exercises 1A and 1B.)									
2A. Alternate grip pull-ups	3	10-8	2-0-1-0						
2B. Barbell shrugs	3	10	2-0-1-1						
2C. Dumbbell lateral raises	3	10	2-0-1-0						
(Rest 2–3 minutes and repeat exercises 2A, 2B, and 2C.)									

Table 10.3 Hard Gainer's Workout, Workout Chart 3

Exercise	Sets	Reps	Tempo	Week 1	Week 2	Week 3	Week 4	Week 5	Week 6
W1. Spidermans	1	20	1-0-1-1	Weights					
W2. One-leg dynamic bridging	1	2 × 12	2-0-1-1						
W3. Plank one-arm reach-outs	1	20	1-1-1-1						
(Once warm-up exercises are completed, begin strength training.)									
1A. Cable two-arm horizontal chest presses	3	12	2-0-1-1						
1B. Dumbbell Zercher squats	3	12	3-0-1-1						
1C. Dips	3	12-15	2-0-1-1						
(Rest 2–3 minutes and repeat exercises 1A, 1B, and 1C.)									
2A. Cable supinated seated rows	3	12	2-01-1						
2B. Dumbbell walking lunges	3	20	2-0-1-0						
2C. Barbell curls		12	2-0-1-1						
(Rest 2–3 minutes and repeat exercises 2A, 2B, and 2C.)									

SPIDERMANS

EXERCISE NOTES

Complete the dynamic warm-up exercises before performing all three weight workouts in the Hard Gainer's Workout.

Start

Step 1: *(a)* Get into a push-up position with your hands on the floor placed just outside shoulder-width apart.

Step 2: Keep your hips raised so that they are parallel to the floor or slightly higher and place your feet hip-width to shoulder-width apart.

Midpoint

Step 3: *(b)* Bend your right knee, lunge your right foot up to your right hand, and place it on the floor beside your hand.

Finish

Step 4: Place your right foot back in the starting position and then repeat the same movement on your left side by bringing your left foot onto the floor beside your left hand.

Step 5: Continue alternating sides for the desired number of reps.

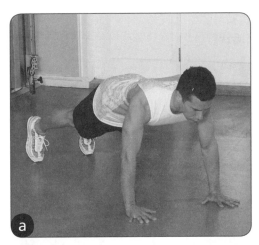

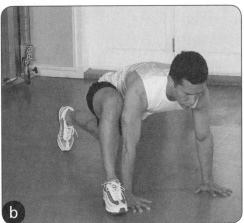

TRAINING TIP

Stretch your hip only as far as it can and then just place your foot on the floor at that stretched position. You may make it only halfway to your hand the first time you try it, but after a few weeks of practicing this movement and stretching, you should see a noticeable improvement in your hip mobility and flexibility.

ONE-LEG DYNAMIC BRIDGING

EXERCISE NOTES

- Complete the dynamic warm-up exercises before performing all three weight workouts in the Hard Gainer's Workout.
- Complete this exercise directly after performing spidermans.

Start

Step 1: Lie on your back.

Step 2: Pull both feet into your hips.

Step 3: Fold your arms across your chest.

Step 4: Keep your knees directly over your ankles and your feet flat on the floor.

Step 5: Engage your glutes by squeezing them together.

Step 6: Lift your right leg straight up in the air and keep it there throughout the set while the left side works.

Midpoint

Step 7: *(a)* Keeping your glutes engaged, exhale, and push your hips off the floor as high as you can lift them without lifting your heel.

Finish

Step 8: *(b)* Slowly breathe in and lower your hips to 1 inch (2.5 cm) above the floor (do not touch the floor).

Step 9: Repeat by lifting and lowering your hips slowly.

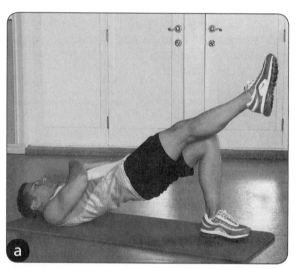

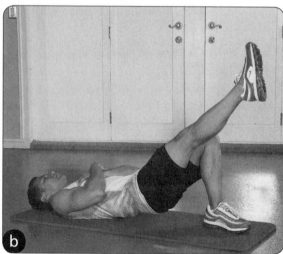

TRAINING TIP

Stay balanced and do not allow your hips or the foot that is in contact with the ground to wobble or tilt to one side. Concentrate on squeezing your glutes!

PLANK ONE-ARM REACH-OUTS

EXERCISE NOTES

- Complete the dynamic warm-up exercises before performing all three weight workouts in the Hard Gainer's Workout.
- Complete this exercise directly after performing one-leg dynamic bridging.

Start

Step 1: *(a)* Get into a plank position with your forearms on the floor directly beneath your shoulders.

Step 2: Keep your hips raised so that they are parallel to the floor or slightly higher and place your feet slightly apart.

Midpoint

Step 3: *(b)* After you feel as if you have engaged your core, lift your left hand off the floor, reach out in front of your left shoulder, and hold your arm out at shoulder height.

Finish

Step 4: Lower your left hand back down onto the floor.

Step 5: Repeat by lifting your right hand off the floor and then bringing that arm in front of your right shoulder as you just did on the left side. Place the right forearm back down on the floor and continue to alternate sides for the desired number of reps.

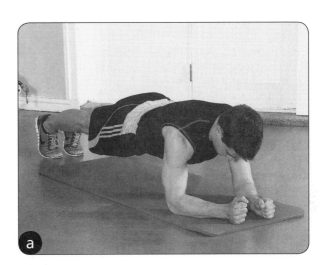

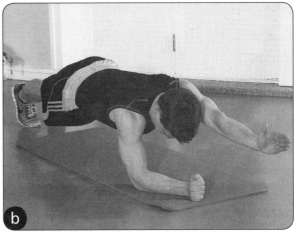

TRAINING TIP

This exercise is easy to cheat on, so make sure that you do not tilt your body to the side where the arm is supporting you as you raise the opposite arm. Keep your back and hips level in a push-up plank position as you stretch your arm straight in front of your shoulder. This exercise is a great way to warm up the upper body and core!

BARBELL INCLINE CHEST PRESSES

EXERCISE NOTES

- Complete the dynamic warm-up exercises first.
- This is the first exercise in the first workout of the Hard Gainer's Workout.

Start

Step 1: Lie back on a 45-degree inclined bench directly under a barbell and plant both feet firmly on the floor.

Step 2: Grip the bar just outside shoulder-width apart and lift it off the bench press rack, holding it directly above your chest.

Midpoint

Step 3: *(a)* Lower the barbell slowly down toward the top of your chest. The bar should stop about 1 to 2 inches (2.5 to 5 cm) above your chest.

Finish

Step 4: *(b)* Exhale as you press the bar above your chest to help produce force and then repeat.

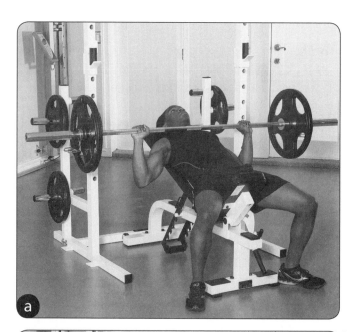

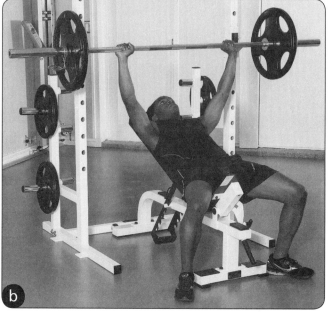

TRAINING TIP

This exercise helps you build up the area between your shoulders and upper chest to create a fuller-looking, more muscular chest. Remember to keep your feet, back, and head in a five-point position at all times.

BARBELL ROMANIAN DEADLIFTS

EXERCISE NOTES

- This is the second exercise in the second superset of the first workout of the Hard Gainer's Workout.
- Complete this exercise directly after performing barbell incline chest presses.
- Because this is the second exercise in your superset, you will rest after completing it.

Start

Step 1: Stand over a barbell with your feet hip-width apart and grip the bar slightly wider than your thighs using an overhand alternate grip (one hand palm facing up and the other palm facing down).

Step 2: *(a)* Maintaining a tight grip, tight core, and neutral spine, pull the bar off the rack and allow it to rest against your quads. Keeping a flat back (neutral spine), retract your shoulder blades and place a slight bend in your knees.

Midpoint

Step 3: *(b)* Allow your hips to stretch backward (with as much as a 20-degree bend in your knees) until you can't stretch your hamstrings and glutes anymore. Your upper body will lower a little, but the hips always move first and dictate how low you go. Do not drop your upper torso toward the floor as you lower the weight just to get deeper into the movement. This action will not provide any more benefit to your legs and may lead to injury.

Finish

Step 4: Squeeze your glutes, push your hips forward, and pull your upper body back to the starting position before performing the next repetition. Exhale as you exert force and lift up.

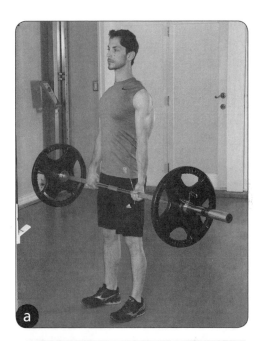

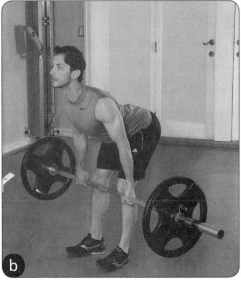

TRAINING TIP

This exercise may be the best way to build muscle in your hamstrings and glutes! Keep your weight way back on your heels and make sure to end the movement when your hips will not stretch back behind you any farther.

BARBELL BENT-OVER ROWS

EXERCISE NOTES

- Complete the entire first superset three or four times before moving on to this second group of exercises.
- This is the first exercise in the second superset of the Hard Gainer's Workout.

Start

Step 1: Stand over a barbell with your feet about shoulder-width apart and grip the bar slightly wider than your thighs using an overhand pronated grip.

Step 2: Using a tight grip, core, and neutral spine, pull the bar off the rack and allow it to rest against your quads.

Step 3: Sit back with your hips into a half squat and allow your upper body to tilt forward with a neutral spine (flat back).

Midpoint

Step 4: *(a)* Holding the bar right in front of your knees, *(b)* retract your shoulder blades and pull your elbows up so that the bar pulls into your abs.

Finish

Step 5: Without allowing your shoulder blades to round out, slowly lower the bar back to the starting position so that the dumbbell ends beside your knees.

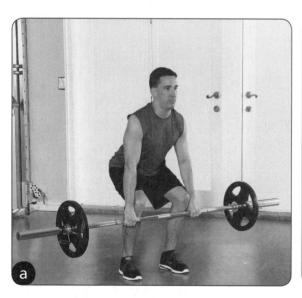 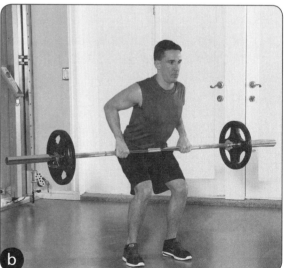

TRAINING TIP

Besides not allowing your back to round or yourself to stand up as you row the weight, focus on not shrugging the weight with your traps and allowing your elbows to flare out to the sides. Instead, keep your elbows close to your body and stay down in your stance so that you can retract your shoulder blades and use your big back muscles to move the weight.

BARBELL FRONT SQUATS

EXERCISE NOTES

- This is the second exercise in the second superset of the third workout of the Hard Gainer's Workout.
- Complete this exercise directly after performing barbell bent-over rows.
- Because this is the second exercise in your superset, you will rest after completing it.

Start

Step 1: Stand with your feet hip-width apart and place a slight bend in your knees.

Step 2: *(a)* Step under the barbell and place it directly on your anterior deltoid and other shoulder muscles so that the bar touches the front of your neck right above your collarbone. (You'll know that the bar is in the right position if you can balance it without touching it with your hands.)

Step 3: Grab the bar either by folding your arms over it and holding it with your hands face down or by using a traditional front squat grip in which you rotate your elbows forward and allow your fingers and wrists to stretch back so that the palms rest on top of your shoulders to hold the bar.

Midpoint

Step 4: Slowly breathe in, keep your chest and elbows lifted high, and sit back with your hips, keeping the weight on your heels.

Step 5: *(b)* Squat as deep as you can without rounding out your lower back, letting your heels come up, allowing your knees to go over your toes, dropping your chest, or going into a posterior pelvic tilt.

Finish

Step 6: Drive hard through your hips and heels to propel yourself back to the standing start position.

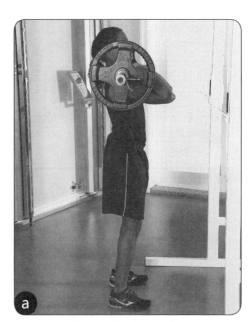

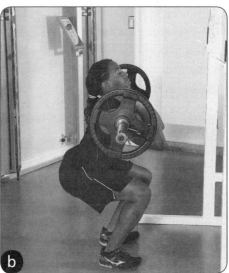

TRAINING TIP

There's a reason that you don't see the average guy doing this exercise—it's hard! But if you can get over the fact that you won't be able to front squat as much as you back squat, you'll be way ahead of the game. This exercise is phenomenal for developing a powerful core (abs) and massive quads!

BARBELL MILITARY SHOULDER PRESSES

EXERCISE NOTES

- Complete the dynamic warm-up exercises first.
- This is the first exercise in the second workout of the Hard Gainer's Workout.

Start

Step 1: *(a)* Stand with your feet shoulder-width apart and hold a barbell with your palms facing away from you slightly wider than shoulder-width at the top of your shoulders.

Step 2: Keep your knees bent and your core engaged throughout the set.

Midpoint

Step 3: *(b)* Press the barbell directly overhead without arching your lower back or tilting your head too far back.

Finish

Step 4: Slowly decelerate the weight back to the starting position above your shoulders while keeping tension on the deltoids.

Step 5: Maintain form and repeat.

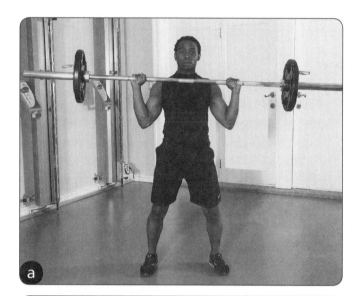

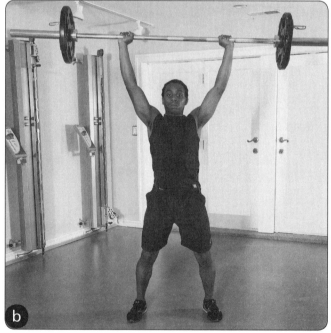

TRAINING TIP

This exercise is a fantastic mass builder for your shoulders, and you'll want to load up the bar with as much weight as you can handle with good form. But you should be conscious throughout the set about not arching your lower back and making sure that you can decelerate the weight back down to the starting position after you lift it overhead.

BARBELL BOX STEP-UPS

EXERCISE NOTES

- This is the second exercise in the Hard Gainer's Workout.
- Complete this exercise directly after performing barbell military shoulder presses.
- Because this is the second exercise in the superset, you will rest before repeating.

Start

Step 1: Place a box or bench that is approximately knee height on the floor in front of you.

Step 2: Step under a barbell and rest it on your trapezius muscles as you would for a back squat. Ensure that your posture remains strong by keeping your shoulder blades pulled back while lifting your chest up.

Step 3: (a) Place your left foot up on the step and leave your right foot on the ground.

Midpoint

Step 4: (b) Keep the weight on your left heel and push up through the left foot and hip until you are standing up straight on top of the box.

Finish

Step 5: Continue to keep your left foot on the box and step back down slowly with your right foot, absorbing the impact so that you can barely hear that foot land. Do not rock backward when you land and keep the weight on the hip and heel of the left leg throughout the set.

Step 6: Complete all your repetitions with the left leg and then switch to the right.

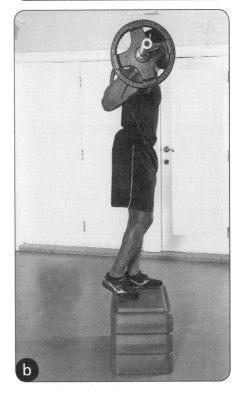

TRAINING TIP

Step-ups not only help build up the muscle in your legs but also can dramatically increase your leg strength and stability. Also, with the barbell now loaded on top of your shoulders, you are getting an intense core-training stimulus!

ALTERNATE GRIP PULL-UPS

EXERCISE NOTES

- Complete the entire first superset three times before moving on to the second group of exercises.
- This is the first exercise in the second tri-set of the second workout in the Hard Gainer's Workout.

Start

Step 1: Grip a straight pull-up (chin-up) bar with your hands shoulder-width apart and have one hand facing away from you and one palm facing toward you.

Step 2: *(a)* Engage your core to prevent yourself from swinging and then lift your legs off the floor by bending your knees. Consider crossing your legs for added stability.

Midpoint

Step 3: *(b)* Using your back muscles (by squeezing your lats and rhomboids), pull yourself up so that your chest comes up to the bar and your forearms touch your biceps.

Finish

Step 4: Slowly lower yourself to the point just before your elbows lock out.

Step 5: Repeat by alternating which hand faces you in next set. You can add weight to increase the difficulty of the exercise so that you can achieve the desired repetition range.

TRAINING TIP

Alternate grip pull-ups are a hybrid exercise that lies somewhere between a chin-up and a pull-up. Therefore, you use slightly more biceps on one side, allowing you to make it slightly easier to do more reps. If you need to use a band for assistance, do so in the beginning. As you gradually build up strength you will be able to switch over to unassisted pull-ups.

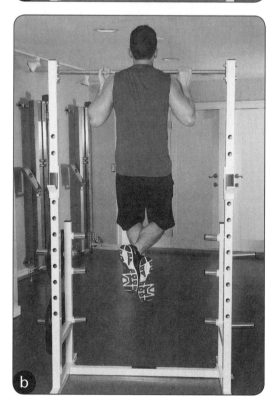

BARBELL SHRUGS

EXERCISE NOTES

- This is the second exercise in the second tri-set of the second workout in the Hard Gainer's Workout.
- Complete this exercise directly after performing alternate grip pull-ups.

Start

Step 1: Place a weighted barbell on a rack just above knee height.

Step 2: Stand over the barbell and place your feet shoulder-width apart.

Step 3: Grip the barbell slightly wider than your hips and have both palms facing you.

Step 4: *(a)* Keeping your core engaged, pull the barbell into your quadriceps, and pull the bar off the rack while maintaining good posture. Your shoulders should not be rounded forward, and your knees should remain slightly bent. Your arms should remain straight throughout the set.

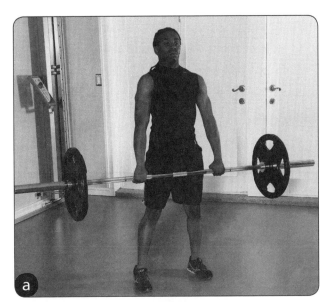

Midpoint

Step 5: *(b)* Look straight ahead throughout the set and shrug your shoulders up as high as you can toward your ears.

Step 6: Hold and squeeze the upper trapezius muscles at the top.

Finish

Step 7: Slowly lower the bar back down your body until your trapezius muscles fully stretch without your rounding your shoulders forward.

Step 8: Repeat.

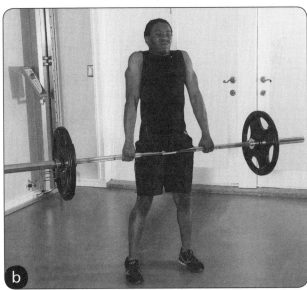

TRAINING TIP

This straightforward exercise allows you to lift the maximum weight possible. The key is to use a full range of motion by trying to touch your shoulders to your ears with each concentric squeeze up with the bar. Although the pull upward with your traps should be fast, the eccentric lowering movement of the bar back to the starting position should be slow and controlled.

DUMBBELL LATERAL RAISES

EXERCISE NOTES

- This is the third exercise in the second tri-set of the second workout in the Hard Gainer's Workout.
- Complete this exercise directly after performing barbell shrugs.
- Because this is the third exercise in the tri-set, you will rest before repeating.

Start

Step 1: *(a)* Stand with your feet hip-width apart and hold two dumbbells to the outside of your legs.

Step 2: Bend your elbows so that they maintain about a 10-degrees angle.

Step 3: Engage your core before lifting the weights so that you do not sway forward or backward.

Midpoint

Step 4: *(b)* Using the muscles of your shoulder, raise the dumbbells up to shoulder height by leading with your upper arm and elbow. Keep the dumbbells in the same plane of motion and do not cheat by moving them in front of your body.

Finish

Step 5: Slowly decelerate the weights back to the starting position while feeling your shoulder muscles stretch. Keep the tension on your shoulders throughout the set and maintain stability in your shoulder joints.

Step 6: Repeat for the desired number of reps.

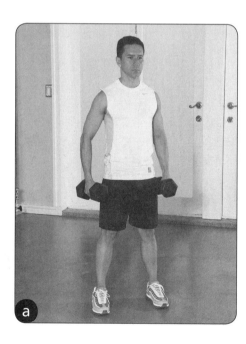 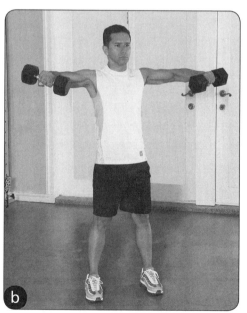

TRAINING TIP

Although I have you do a few single-joint exercises, this one is fantastic for improving rotator cuff stability and strength. This movement also is great for building bulk to the outsides of your shoulders, leading to a fuller and broader look for your upper body. Keep in mind that the less you bend your elbows in this exercise, the more you force your shoulders to do the work.

CABLE TWO-ARM HORIZONTAL CHEST PRESSES

EXERCISE NOTES

- Complete the dynamic warm-up exercises first.
- This is the first exercise in the third workout of the Hard Gainer's Workout.

Start

Step 1: Grab two cable handles attached at shoulder height.

Step 2: *(a)* Step forward with either leg into a staggered stance and remain there throughout the set.

Step 3: Point your palms to face the floor and keep your wrists, elbows, and shoulders on the same plane.

Midpoint

Step 4: *(b)* Press the cables out and forcefully squeeze your pectorals and the handles together. Exhale at this point to help produce force.

Finish

Step 5: Slowly decelerate the weight back to the starting position while feeling your chest and shoulder muscles stretch. Keep the tension on your chest throughout the set and maintain a strong balanced stance.

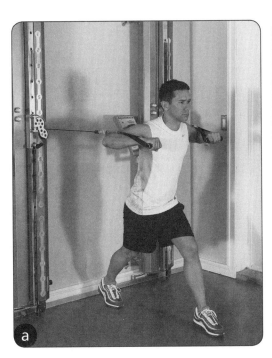
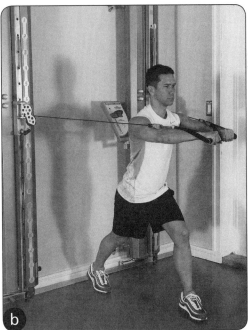

TRAINING TIP

By using both arms you will be able to increase stability in your core and thus push more weight. Make sure to position your body as upright as possible and remember not to overextend your shoulders while pressing at chest height.

DUMBBELL ZERCHER SQUATS

EXERCISE NOTES

- This is the second exercise in first tri-set of the third Hard Gainer's Workout.
- Complete this exercise directly after performing cable two-arm horizontal chest presses.

Start

Step 1: Hold a single heavy dumbbell on your biceps by wrapping your forearms and hands around it in a modified Zercher hold.

Step 2: *(a)* Keep the dumbbell held up high in front of your chest.

Step 3: Place your weight back on your heels and maintain a shoulder-width stance.

Midpoint

Step 4: *(b)* Keeping your core engaged sit back with your hips into a deep squat while maintaining good posture and keeping your chest up.

Finish

Step 5: Drive through your heels while exhaling and push your body back to a standing position. Do not move the dumbbell from in front of your chest throughout the set.

Step 6: Repeat.

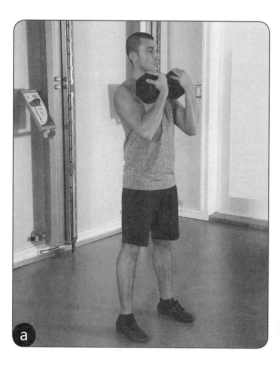 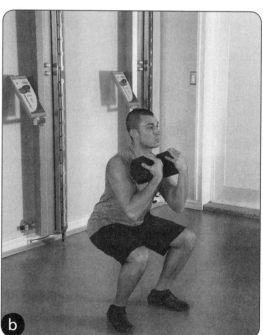

TRAINING TIP

Keep the weight back on your heels and do not allow your knees to cheat forward over your toes. Also, try not to curl the dumbbell, but rather make it a part of your upper body and use your core to hold yourself upright.

DIPS

EXERCISE NOTES

- This is the third exercise in the third workout of the Hard Gainer's Workout.
- Complete this exercise directly after performing dumbbell Zercher squats.
- Because this is the third exercise in your tri-set, you will rest after completing it.

Start

Step 1: Using parallel bar dip handles, grip both sides and tilt your chest slightly forward.

Step 2: *(a)* Hold yourself up in the air and lift your legs off the ground.

Step 3: Keeping your elbows in alignment with your shoulders (do not allow them to flare out) slowly lower yourself down.

Midpoint

Step 4: *(b)* Stop when your biceps are parallel to the ground or just above that point if you are feeling unstable or tight through your shoulders.

Finish

Step 5: Squeeze your triceps while straightening your elbows and pushing yourself to the starting position.

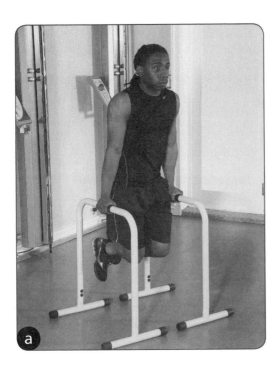
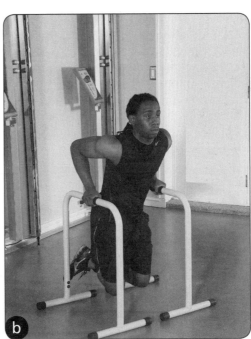

TRAINING TIP

I'm a huge fan of dips for triceps, shoulder, and chest development, but you must be careful to keep the tension on those muscles all the way through the movement. Be sure not to stretch too deep and cause too much shoulder flexion.

CABLE SUPINATED SEATED ROWS

EXERCISE NOTES

- Complete the entire first tri-three times before moving on to the second group of exercises.
- This is the first exercise in the second tri-set of the third Hard Gainer's Workout.

Start

Step 1: *(a)* Affix a straight lat bar attachment to a seated row machine and grip it hip-width apart using an underhand supinated grip while seated on the bench.

Step 2: With your knees bent, place both feet against the footrest, engage your core, and retract your shoulder blades.

Step 3: Push back with both legs to your starting position while maintaining a neutral spine and good posture. Keep your knees slightly bent throughout the set.

Midpoint

Step 4: *(b)* Concentrate on squeezing your shoulder blades back while stretching open your chest as you complete your first repetition by pulling the bar into your navel and abdomen.

Finish

Step 5: Without allowing your shoulder blades or back to round forward, return your arms back to their extended starting position. Maintain tension on your back muscles at all times.

Step 6: Repeat for the desired number of reps.

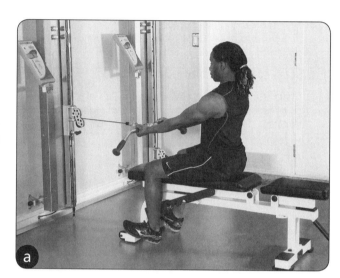

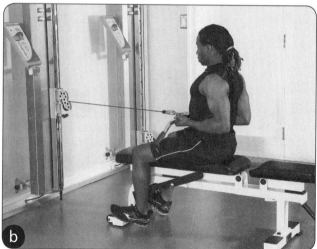

TRAINING TIP

This supinated seated row movement will enable you to pull some serious weight while using both your larger back muscles and your smaller arm muscles like the forearms and biceps. As always when you're doing a seated row, make sure not to round out your back as you're returning the weight to the cable weight stack with each rep.

DUMBBELL WALKING LUNGES

EXERCISE NOTES

- This is the second exercise in the second tri-set of the third Hard Gainer's Workout.
- Complete this exercise directly after performing cable supinated seated rows.

Start

Step 1: *(a)* Grab a pair of heavy dumbbells and hold them by your sides.

Step 2: Pull your shoulder blades back and keep them retracted for the remainder of the set.

Step 3: Step forward with one leg, keeping your weight on the heel of that foot.

Midpoint

Step 4: *(b)* Sit into the hip of the front leg as you lower your back knee into a lunge.

Step 5: Continue to keep the weight on your front hip and heel as you push up through them to propel yourself back to the top.

Finish

Step 6: Step together with both feet or step forward with the back leg as you come to the top of your stance.

Step 7: Repeat by alternating sides.

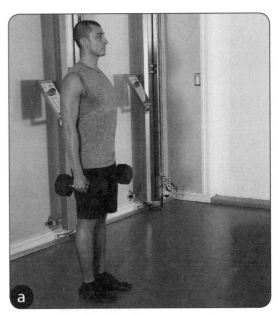

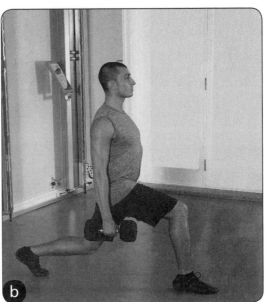

TRAINING TIP

You should take a step large enough that you can sit into your front hip and heel without allowing your front knee to go over your toes. This movement also activates the glute muscles to a greater degree.

BARBELL CURLS

EXERCISE NOTES

- This is the third exercise in the second tri-set of the third workout of the Hard Gainer's Workout.
- Complete this exercise directly after performing dumbbell walking lunges.
- Because this is the third exercise in your tri-set, you will rest after completing it.

Start

Step 1: *(a)* Stand with your feet hip-width apart and hold a barbell about 1 inch (2.5 cm) in front of your quadriceps.

Step 2: Keep your chest up, shoulder blades retracted, knees bent, and chin parallel to the ground throughout the set. Moving just your forearms, curl the bar up toward your chest.

Midpoint

Step 3: *(b)* Squeeze your biceps forcefully until your forearms touch your biceps. Do not allow your elbows to pull forward or your shoulder blades to round.

Finish

Step 4: Slowly allow the weight to return to the starting position by allowing your elbows to straighten back down.

Step 5: Before your biceps and forearms lose tension, begin your next repetition.

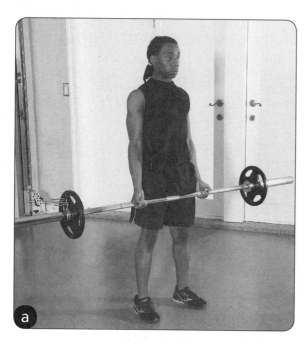 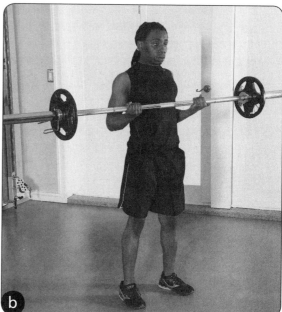

TRAINING TIP

The biggest mistake I see with barbell curls is allowing the elbows to come away from the sides, which permits the bar to come all the way up to the collarbone or neck. This action decreases the amount of tension on the biceps and allows them to rest to a certain extent. To increase the tension, you should use your elbows as your fulcrum and pull them back to allow your forearms to be the lever that moves the weight.

CHAPTER 11

Functional Training Workout

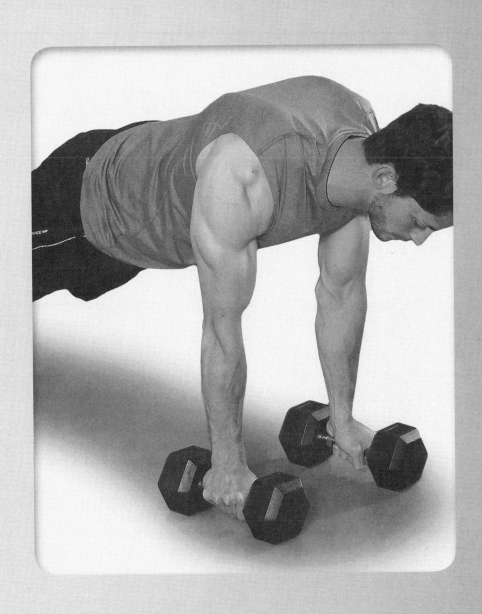

I've mentioned this in a previous chapter, but it's worth repeating.

Functional training is not standing on a stability ball or trying to juggle dumbbells while touching your nose. The term *functional training* has been widely misused to refer to any type of exercise that forces your body to perform some type of stabilization-based exercise.

Many of these movements, however, are far removed from how your body functions and reacts in space. Therefore, many of the so-called functional movements are just made-up, unsafe exercises.

We're going to concentrate the Functional Training Workout program on training like an athlete to develop speed, power, strength, and agility, all while building off previous functionally based movement patterns.

The exercises in this six-week program will challenge your core in a whole new way. We're going to take your training to the next level here.

You're going to find some movements that you may have already tried before, but now we're putting a whole new twist on them. You'll be using some kettlebells and even a landmine (I'll explain later).

In addition, each of the three unique workouts targets your body in a slightly different way using complementary movement pairings and repetition schemes. By changing how your body must adapt to each new exercise, we're constantly forcing it to become stronger and more powerful (slowly progressing up in weight each week). Make sure to use table 11.1 and tables 11.2 and 11.3 on page 194 as a basis to track your workouts.

Lastly, if you've ever wondered how some men's fitness models and athletes look as if they have abs on top of their abs, I'll share their secret with you. Trust me when I tell you how the pros create that rock-hard, yet highly functional physique.

Those striated, charcoal-briquette-looking abs, obliques, and serratus anterior muscles (the cool-looking muscles under the arms and over the ribs) aren't created by crunches alone.

A well-defined midsection is the result of working the core muscles through a multitude of exercises that require maximal contraction during heavy lifts, rotational movements, and deep isometric holds.

You need to train like an athlete to look like one.

And that's just what we're going to do in this program. You're about to begin challenging your body in every way possible to develop a functional, lean, and fit physique. It's the kind of body that you can be proud of showing off at home, in the gym, at the beach, or maybe out on the playing field!

Top 10 Tips and Benefits of the Functional Training Workout:

1. Start off light and learn each new movement.

2. Remember that it takes more than crunches to get a great-looking six-pack. In this program you'll be targeting your core in every way possible to create a stronger, more powerful midsection.

3. Because we now know that functional training is more than just standing on a stability ball, I've designed a six-week program that will help you develop full-body functional strength. Your legs, arms, and core will be much more powerful by the end of week 6.

4. Although I have outlined a few kettlebell movements that I would like you to complete as part of this program, you can always substitute a dumbbell in their place if you don't have access to kettlebells.

5. Be sure to study the photo and exercise demonstration before you attempt a movement. I suggest that you take this book to the gym to refer to during your workouts.

6. As with any program in which you are looking to make muscular and strength adaptations, you should aim to increase the amount of weight that you lift each week (without compromising form, of course).

7. I handpicked each exercise when I designed these programs, so it's best not to substitute any exercise for another.

8. Remember that the exercises that are most challenging for you (usually the ones that you don't like) are often the ones that you need the most because they typically reveal a weakness in your body.

9. You'll find that the first and second weeks are the hardest because you're adapting to the new movement patterns. By week 3, however, you're going to feel stronger and more energized.

10. By the end of the Functional Training Workout routine you should find that your body and core have never felt stronger or tighter!

Table 11.1 Functional Training Workout, Workout Chart 1

Exercise	Sets	Reps	Tempo	Week 1	Week 2	Week 3	Week 4	Week 5	Week 6
W1. Inchworms	1	20	1-0-1-1			Weights			
W2. Stick overhead squats	1	12	2-0-1-0						
W3. Vertical frog jumps	1	10	0						
(Once warm-up exercises are completed, begin strength training.)									
1A. Barbell one-arm squat presses	3	2 x 10	2-0-1-1						
1B. Dumbbell Zercher step-ups	3	20	2-0-1-0						
1C. Oblique twists (slams)	3	2 x 12-15	1-0-1-0						
(Rest 2–3 minutes and repeat exercises 1A, 1B, and 1C.)									
2A. Dumbbell renegade rows	3	24-30	2-0-1-0						
2B. Dumbbell Bulgarian split squats	3	2 x 12	3-0-1-1						
2C. Kettlebell alternating one-arm swings	3	20	1-0-1-0						
(Rest 2–3 minutes and repeat exercises 2A, 2B, and 2C.)									

Table 11.2 Functional Training Workout, Workout Chart 2

Exercise	Sets	Reps	Tempo	Week 1	Week 2	Week 3	Week 4	Week 5	Week 6
W1. Inchworms	1	20	1-0-1-1	Weights					
W2. Stick overhead squats	1	12	2-0-1-0						
W3. Vertical frog jumps	1	10	0						
(Once warm-up exercises are completed, begin strength training.)									
1A. Cable push–pulls	3	2 x 12	1-0-1-0						
1B. Barbell overhead forward lunges	3	20	2-0-1-0						
(Rest 2–3 minutes and repeat exercises 1A and 1B.)									
2A. Dumbbell goblet squats	3	12-10	3-0-1-0						
2B. Turkish half get-ups	3	2 x 8-10	1-0-1-1						
(Rest 2–3 minutes and repeat exercises 2A and 2B.)									
3A. Stability ball pikes	3	AMAP (15-20)	2-0-1-0						
3B. Stability ball back reverse extensions	3	15	2-0-1-1						
(Rest 2–3 minutes and repeat exercises 3A and 3B.)									

Table 11.3 Functional Training Workout, Workout Chart 3

Exercise	Sets	Reps	Tempo	Week 1	Week 2	Week 3	Week 4	Week 5	Week 6
W1. Inchworms	1	20	1-0-1-1	Weights					
W2. Stick overhead squats	1	12	2-0-1-0						
W3. Vertical frog jumps	1	10	0						
(Once warm-up exercises are completed, begin strength training.)									
1A. Kettlebell cleans, front squats, and presses	3	10-8							
1B. Dumbbell one-arm deadlifts from floor	3	2 x 8-5	2-0-1-1						
1C. Hanging knee-ups	3	AMAP (15-20)	2-0-1-0						
(Rest 2–3 minutes and repeat exercises 1A, 1B, and 1C.)									
2A. Barbell supinated inverted rows	3	AMAP (15-20)	2-0-1-1						
2B. Barbell shoulder-loaded walking lunges	3	16-20	2-0-1-0						
2C. Kettlebell two-arm swings	3	8-10	1-0-1-0						
(Rest 2–3 minutes and repeat exercises 2A, 2B, and 2C.)									

INCHWORMS

EXERCISE NOTES

Complete the dynamic warm-up exercises first before performing all three weight workouts in the Functional Training Workout.

Start

Step 1: Stand with your feet together.

Step 2: *(a)* Place both hands directly on the floor in front of your feet.

Step 3: Keep your fingers and palms in contact with the ground throughout the set and begin walking each hand out, one after another.

Midpoint

Step 4: *(b)* Make sure to keep your core engaged throughout the set so that you do not let your hips drop toward the floor. Walk your hands out past the push-up position if possible and stay on the balls of your feet.

Step 5: After you have walked your hands out as far as you can, begin to make small steps with your legs and walk your feet into your hands. Try to keep your knees straight and walk in only as far as your lower back and hamstrings will allow.

Finish

Step 6: After you have walked your feet in as far as you can to your hands, begin to walk your hands back out as far as you can and repeat the process. When you do inchworms correctly you will be walking your hands out and then walking your feet in with each rep to move forward down the floor.

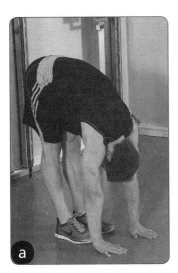
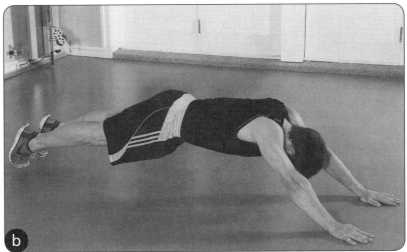

TRAINING TIP

Besides giving your backside a great stretch, you get to warm up your shoulders and core with this fantastic movement. Remember to keep your fingers and palms in contact with the ground throughout the set.

STICK OVERHEAD SQUATS

EXERCISE NOTES

- Complete the dynamic warm-up exercises first before performing all three weight workouts in the Functional Training Workout.
- Complete this exercise directly after performing inchworms.

Start

Step 1: *(a)* Hold a wooden dowel or light bar wider than shoulder-width apart and raise it above your head. Stand with your feet shoulder-width apart and allow your hips to sit back slightly.

Step 2: Let the stick stretch open your chest and keep your elbows straight as the bar locks back into position behind your head. Your shoulder blades should be pulled back for support. The stick should not move from this position throughout the set.

Midpoint

Step 3: *(b)* Inhale and sit back into a squat, allowing the weight to fall back onto your heels.

Step 4: Continue to keep your chest up, look straight ahead, and keep your chin parallel to the floor.

Finish

Step 5: Drive through your heels and hips to propel yourself back to your standing position.

Step 6: Repeat.

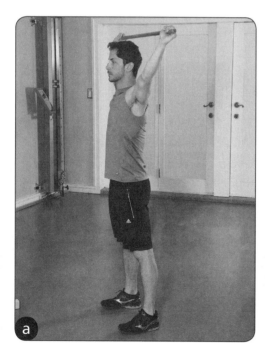
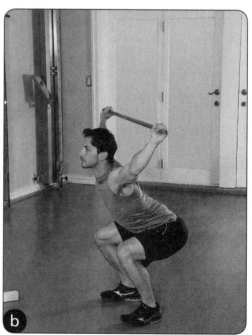

TRAINING TIP

Make sure not to let your knees begin the movement by improperly shifting forward; sit back into your hips instead. To get more comfortable with the movement, I suggest putting a box or bench behind you to learn to sit back into the squat.

VERTICAL FROG JUMPS

EXERCISE NOTES

- Complete the dynamic warm-up exercises first before performing all three weight workouts in the Functional Training Workout.
- Complete this exercise directly after performing stick overhead squats.

Start

Step 1: *(a)* Squat down as low as you can and press your fingers against the ground between your legs.

Step 2: Keep your chest up and maintain your balance.

Midpoint

Step 3: *(b)* Next, jump as high as you can straight up while raising your arms above your head.

Finish

Step 4: Land softly on the floor with your legs bending back into a squat and immediately go into your next repetition while maintaining proper form.

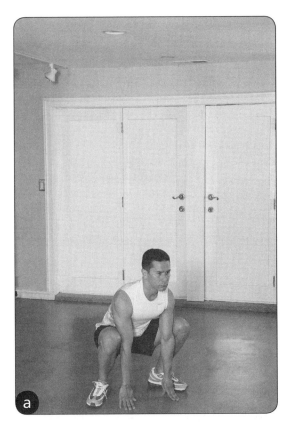
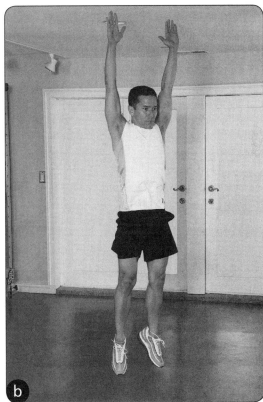

TRAINING TIP

You're going to get a great stretch through your upper hamstrings, hips, and glutes. At the same time you'll be firing your nervous system and forcing your muscles to move at maximum speed to propel your arms up into the air with each jump. Try to stretch your body fully by reaching overhead on the jump and then absorbing the impact on the way down.

BARBELL ONE-ARM SQUAT PRESSES

EXERCISE NOTES

- Complete the dynamic warm-up exercises first.
- This is the first exercise in the first workout of the Functional Training Workout.

Start

Step 1: Place a barbell on the floor in a corner where two walls meet or into a device called a landmine (it looks like home plate with a cylinder attached to it to place the bar into).

Step 2: After placing a weight plate on the barbell hold the barbell up in the air at about a 45-degree angle from the ground or slightly higher.

Step 3: Make sure to grip the barbell with your right hand at about the top of the barbell.

Step 4: Keep your knees slightly bent at the top and your core engaged throughout the set.

Midpoint

Step 5: (a) Keeping your chest up and your head looking straight ahead, simultaneously squat down and lower the barbell to about 2 inches (5 cm) above your right shoulder as you reach the bottom of your squat.

Finish

Step 6: (b) Quickly drive through your heels and hips and thrust your entire body and arm back up to the starting position while raising your right arm above your right shoulder into a shoulder press.

Step 7: Repeat all reps on your right side and then switch sides.

TRAINING TIP

This movement is an intense core, shoulder, and leg exercise. Your body has to fight not to twist or rotate on the way down and as you're pressing overhead. Also, keep your free arm off to the side and not helping to support your core by holding onto your hips.

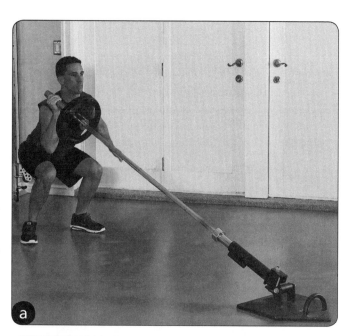

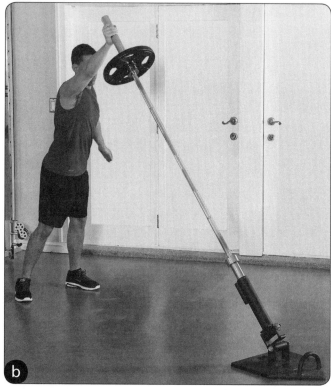

DUMBBELL ZERCHER STEP-UPS

EXERCISE NOTES

- This is the second exercise in the second tri-set of the first workout of the Functional Training Workout.
- Complete this exercise directly after performing barbell one-arm squat presses.

Start

Step 1: Place a box or bench that is approximately knee height on the floor in front of you.

Step 2: Hold a single dumbbell in front of your chest and grip both ends on your biceps by wrapping your hands around each side. You should keep your chest held high and your core engaged so that your back doesn't round forward at any time.

Step 3: *(a)* Place your left foot up on the step and leave your right foot on the ground.

Midpoint

Step 4: *(b)* Keep the weight on your left heel and push up through the foot and hip until you are standing up straight on top of the box.

Finish

Step 5: Keeping your right foot on the box, step down with your left leg. Do not rock backward when you land; keep the weight on the top (right) leg that is up on the box.

Step 6: Repeat by alternating legs and stepping up until you reach the desired number of repetitions.

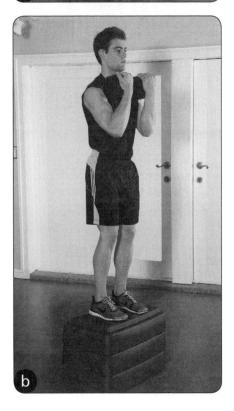

TRAINING TIP

Step-ups have to be one of the most functional exercises in the world because all of us encounter stairs at some point almost every day. If we can do step-ups holding a 50- or 60-pound (23 or 27 kg) dumbbell, 10 flights of regular stairs will feel like a walk in the park! Remember to push through the heel and hip of the leg that is up on the box. Also, make sure not to rock back onto the back leg as it steps off the box.

OBLIQUE TWISTS (SLAMS)

EXERCISE NOTES

- This is the third exercise in the first tri-set of the first workout of the Functional Training Workout.
- Complete this exercise directly after performing dumbbell Zercher step-ups.
- Because this is the third exercise in the first tri-set, you will rest after completing it.

Start

Step 1: Sit on the floor or a padded mat holding a weight plate or medicine ball.

Step 2: Sit back slightly and raise both legs off the ground so that only your hips are in contact with the floor. Keep your core engaged so that you do not round out your back.

Step 3: *(a)* Bring the medicine ball down beside your right hip but do not allow it to touch the floor.

Midpoint

Step 4: *(b)* Keeping yourself stable and balanced, forcefully chop the medicine ball from low beside your right hip to high above your left shoulder. (If you have a partner have him put his hand or a pad above your left shoulder so that you can slam the medicine ball or weight up into the object; this action will force your core to work harder against the reactive forces.)

Finish

Step 5: Slowly return the weight down low beside your right hip but don't let it touch the floor.

Step 6: Repeat on the same side for all repetitions and then switch sides without letting your feet touch.

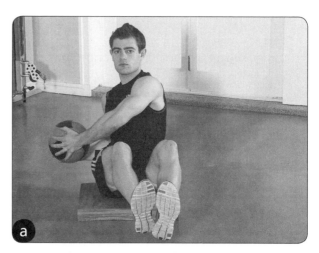

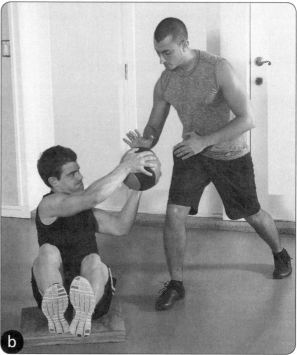

TRAINING TIP

This exercise may seem easy and straightforward, but the movement is challenging, especially if you try not to let your legs swing back and forth as you chop across your body. If you feel any lower back pain or you begin to round out your back, readjust your form or discontinue the movement for that set.

DUMBBELL RENEGADE ROWS

EXERCISE NOTES

- Complete the dynamic warm-up exercises first.
- This is the first exercise in the second workout of the Functional Training Workout.

Start

Step 1: *(a)* Place two dumbbells shoulder-width apart on the floor and get into a push-up position, holding a dumbbell in each hand.

Step 2: Keep your hips up and your feet no more than shoulder-width apart.

Midpoint

Step 3: *(b)* Keeping your core engaged, lift the right dumbbell off the floor by rowing it up using your back muscles behind your right shoulder. Pull the dumbbell toward your right oblique by lifting your elbow high above your back.

Step 4: Slowly lower the weight and place the right dumbbell back on the ground directly below your right shoulder.

Step 5: Repeat this same rowing movement on your left side by lifting that dumbbell off the floor and rowing up to your left oblique area.

Finish

Step 6: Slowly lower the left dumbbell and place it directly beneath your left shoulder.

Step 7: Repeat by alternating sides with each repetition.

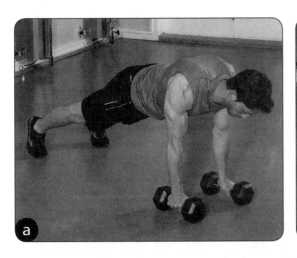 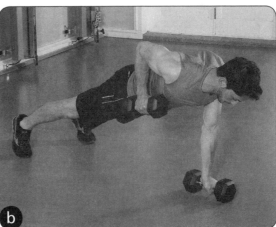

TRAINING TIP

This movement pushes your core, shoulders, back, and pretty much every other muscle in your upper body to the limit. Make sure not to lean or rock to the opposite side of the dumbbell that is being lifted to counterbalance yourself—use your core to do that!

DUMBBELL BULGARIAN SPLIT SQUATS

EXERCISE NOTES

- This is the second exercise in the second tri-set of the first workout of the Functional Training Workout.
- Complete this exercise directly performing after dumbbell renegade rows.

Start

Step 1: Place a box or bench that is approximately knee height on the floor behind you.

Step 2: Hold two dumbbells on your shoulders so that they remain balanced there throughout the set. Use your core to keep your chest up and back in alignment.

Step 3: *(a)* Stand about 3 feet (90 cm) away from the bench and place the top of your right foot on the bench so that your ankle has room to move. You should now be standing on just your left foot.

Midpoint

Step 4: *(b)* Keeping the weight on your left heel and hip, sit back into those areas as you squat or lunge down until your back knee stretches down to just above the floor. (Your legs should resemble close to right angles at this point.)

Finish

Step 5: Push up through your left hip and heel as you stand back up to the starting position, still balancing on just your left leg.

Step 6: Repeat all reps on your left leg and then switch sides.

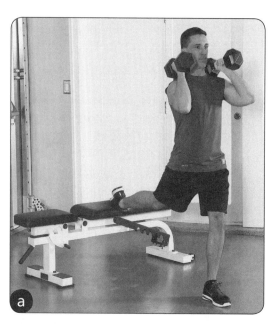
a

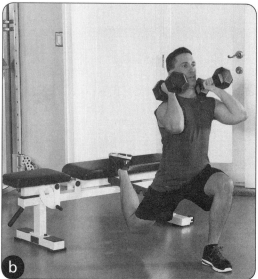
b

TRAINING TIP

Bulgarian slit squats are really a lunge-based movement and thus target similar muscles. You should feel a stretch down the quadriceps and hip flexors of the leg that is on the bench, but the front leg should be the one that is working to take the weight. Allow the back leg to take little weight and instead use it just to keep you balanced.

KETTLEBELL ALTERNATING ONE-ARM SWINGS

EXERCISE NOTES

- This is the third exercise in the second tri-set of the first workout of the Functional Training Workout.
- Complete this exercise directly after performing dumbbell Bulgarian split squats.
- Because this is the third exercise in the tri-set, you will rest after completing it.

Start

Step 1: *(a)* Hold a kettlebell (or dumbbell) between your legs in just your left hand.

Step 2: Keep your spine neutral while sitting back with your hips so that you can feel your hamstrings and glutes stretch.

Step 3: Pretend that you're passing the kettlebell through your legs behind you as you stretch back with your hips.

Midpoint

Step 4: Drive forward and up with your hips to propel yourself to a standing position, allowing the kettlebell to swing up and through your legs.

Step 5: *(b)* As the kettlebell becomes weightless around chest height, switch hands in midair.

Finish

Step 6: Now use your right hand to hold the kettlebell as it swings down between your legs. Go immediately into your next repetition.

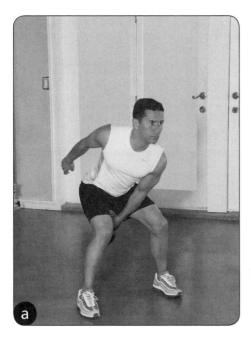
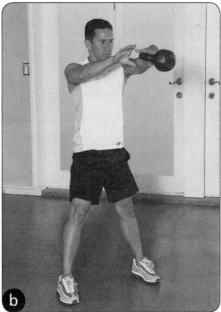

TRAINING TIP

Although you can hold a dumbbell vertically with one hand gripping the handle, the best way to do this exercise is with a kettlebell. Be sure not to swing the weight with your arms but rather use your hips to generate enough power to swing the weight up to about chest height.

CABLE PUSH–PULLS

EXERCISE NOTES

- Complete the dynamic warm-up exercises first.
- This is the first exercise in the second workout of the Functional Training Workout.

Start

Step 1: Attach two cable handles at shoulder height on a cable tower.

Step 2: Face toward your left side and use your right hand (inside arm) to hold the cable attachment that is away from the direction in which you are facing.

Step 3: Use your left hand (outside arm) to grab the handle that is closer to you and positioned directly in front of you.

Step 4: *(a)* Face your hips and shoulders forward toward the cable attachment that your left hand is holding.

Midpoint

Step 5: *(b)* Keep your core engaged and press your right hand forward to complete a chest press while simultaneously pulling your left arm back to do a one-arm horizontal pronated row using your back muscles. Both movements should remain at shoulder height, and you should not twist your body.

Finish

Step 6: Slowly return your arms to their starting position without taking the tension off the cables or allowing your body to rotate.

Step 7: Repeat for the desired number of reps and then turn your body toward your right arm on the inside without letting go of the handles. You will now be facing the other direction and can complete the same movement by pressing on the inside with your left arm and rowing on the outside with your right arm.

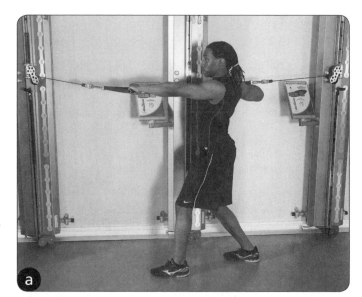

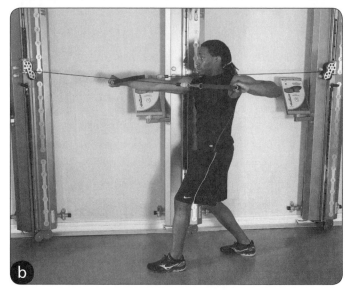

TRAINING TIP

Although this exercise may seem complicated, after you give it a shot you'll find out how quickly you can pick it up. My big tip is to keep your arms on the same plane at shoulder height without allowing your body to rotate. Stick with this one because it's an amazing exercise that targets every muscle of your core and upper body!

BARBELL OVERHEAD FORWARD LUNGES

EXERCISE NOTES

- This is the second exercise in the second superset of the second workout of the Functional Training Workout.
- Complete this exercise directly after performing cable push–pulls.
- Because this is the second exercise in your superset, you will rest after completing it.

Start

Step 1: *(a)* Hold a barbell wider than shoulder-width apart and raise it overhead so that it stretches slightly behind your head.

Step 2: Take a big step forward and land with the heel of your left foot.

Step 3: Sit back with your left hip and allow your right knee to bend down toward the ground.

Midpoint

Step 4: *(b)* Breathe in as your right knee stretches toward the floor and make sure that your left knee stays behind your left toes as you sit back into your left hip and heel. (Your legs should resemble two right angles at the bottom.)

Step 5: Drive back up to the starting position by pushing through your left leg from the bottom position and backward toward your right foot while exhaling.

Finish

Step 6: Keep the bar overhead and steady throughout the set. Stand up tall at the finish with your shoulders pulled back and down.

Step 7: Repeat the process by stepping forward with your right leg and continue alternating sides.

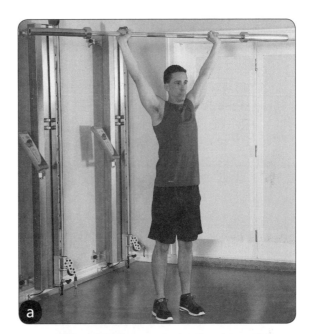

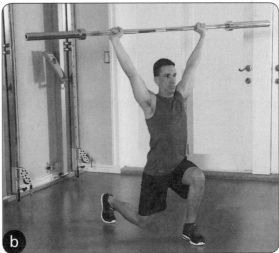

TRAINING TIP

This big-boy exercise will challenge your core and entire body as you struggle to maintain balance and stability with each rep. You'll also receive a full range-of-motion stretch at the bottom of each rep. Focus on keeping the bar stable overhead by locking your arms into position and then not moving them throughout the set.

DUMBBELL GOBLET SQUATS

EXERCISE NOTES

- Complete the entire first superset three times before moving on to the second group of exercises.
- This is the first exercise in the second tri-set of the second workout in the Functional Training Workout.

Start

Step 1: *(a)* Grab a single heavy dumbbell and cup your hands under the head of the dumbbell so that you're holding it up in front of your chest.

Step 2: Keep the dumbbell held up high in front of your chest throughout the set without lowering it on the way down.

Step 3: Place your weight back on your heels and maintain a shoulder-width stance.

Midpoint

Step 4: *(b)* Keeping your core engaged, sit back with your hips into a deep squat while maintaining good posture and keeping your chest up.

Finish

Step 5: Drive through your heels while exhaling and push your body back to a standing position.

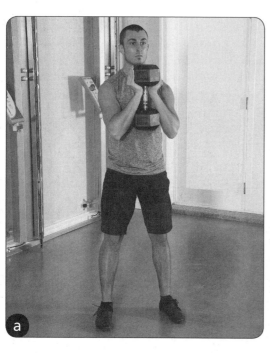
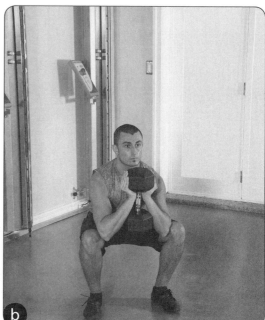

TRAINING TIP

Keep the weight back on your heels and do not allow your knees to cheat forward over your toes. Remember to focus on keeping your core tight so that you don't lean forward or back!

TURKISH HALF GET-UPS

EXERCISE NOTES

- This is the second exercise in the second superset of the second workout of the Functional Training Workout.
- Complete this exercise directly after performing dumbbell goblet squats.
- Because this is the second exercise in your superset, you will rest after completing it.

Start

Step 1: Place a kettlebell on the ground next to the left side of where you will be lying flat on your back.

Step 2: Lie on a mat on your back and then roll toward your left side to grab the kettlebell in your left hand and press it up above your left chest and shoulder (it should remain there throughout the set).

Step 3: (a) Bring your left heel into your left glute and hip and keep your right leg extended out straight.

Step 4: Place your right arm on the floor at a 45-degree angle to the side of your body and have your palm facing down. You will lean into this arm as you lift your upper body to the top.

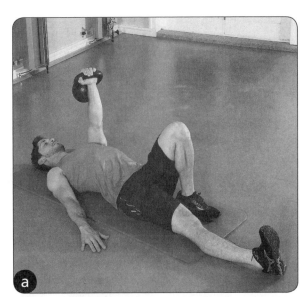

Midpoint

Step 5: (b) Keeping the kettlebell pointed to the sky, lift your upper body off the floor using your abs and core. At the top you should be sitting straight up with your abdomen and chest pulled into your left quad and the kettlebell pointing directly up above your left shoulder.

Finish

Step 6: Keeping your core engaged, slowly decelerate your upper body back down toward the floor without rounding your spine.

Step 7: Complete all your repetitions with the left side and then switch sides.

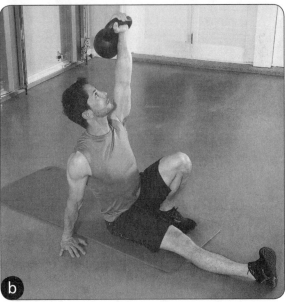

TRAINING TIP

Here are a few must-do tips: (1) Look up at the kettlebell the whole way up and down; (2) do not round your spine at any time; (3) pretend that the kettlebell is a bucket of water that you do not want to spill forward or backward during any part of the movement.

STABILITY BALL PIKES

EXERCISE NOTES

- Complete the entire first and second supersets three times before moving on to the third group of exercises.
- This is the first exercise in the third superset of the second workout in the Functional Training Workout.

Start

Step 1: Start by placing a stability ball under your belly and lying over it in a push-up position.

Step 2: *(a)* Walk your hands all the way out until only your feet and shins are resting on top of the stability ball. Maintain a strong push-up position and do not let your hips sag toward the floor.

Midpoint

Step 3: *(b)* Without moving your arms, pull your hips high into the air and stretch your hamstrings (into a pike) until they are well above your head and shoulders. You should keep your abs pulled in and your core engaged. Your feet will also roll up onto the toes at the peak.

Finish

Step 4: Slowly roll your legs back out to the starting position without shifting your shoulders from above your hands or letting your hips drop below parallel to the ground.

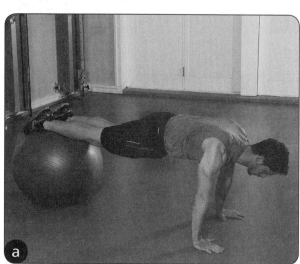 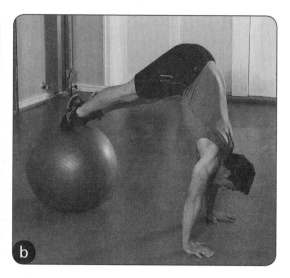

TRAINING TIP

The key to this exercise is to concentrate on your abs and feel them helping you to pull the ball in toward your shoulders on the way up with your hips. Use your core and obliques to prevent you from rolling from side to side and to keep your body steady. After you master this movement you will enjoy greater shoulder and core stability!

STABILITY BALL BACK REVERSE EXTENSIONS

EXERCISE NOTES

- This is the second exercise in the third superset of the second workout of the Functional Training Workout.
- Complete this exercise directly after performing stability ball pikes.
- Because this is the second exercise in your superset, you will rest after completing it.

Start

Step 1: Place a stability ball under your belly and hips.

Step 2: Place both hands under your shoulders in a push-up position.

Step 3: Make sure that you are able to touch only your toes down to the ground behind you.

Midpoint

Step 4: *(a)* Squeeze your glutes and lift both legs off the ground as one unit. Your legs should lift above hip height, and your arms should support you so that you do not dip your upper body into a push-up (your arms are counterbalancing you).

Step 5: Hold and squeeze your lower back and glutes at the top when your legs are at their highest point.

Finish

Step 6: *(b)* Slowly lower your legs down toward the floor but make sure to stop before your feet touch the floor.

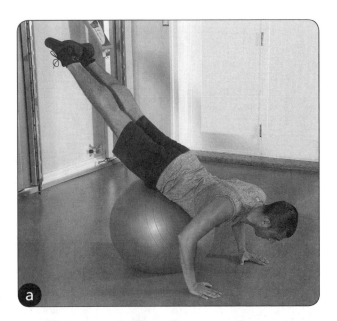

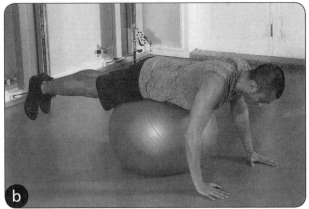

TRAINING TIP

The most common error with this movement is bouncing on the ball to lift the legs back up in the air on each rep. You also want to ensure that you don't let your face come to close to the ground by countering each lift of your legs with your upper body and arms. When done correctly, this exercise is a great complement to your abs exercises and will help balance out your core strength.

KETTLEBELL CLEANS, FRONT SQUATS, AND PRESSES

EXERCISE NOTES

- Complete the dynamic warm-up exercises first.
- This is the first exercise in the third workout of the Functional Training Workout.

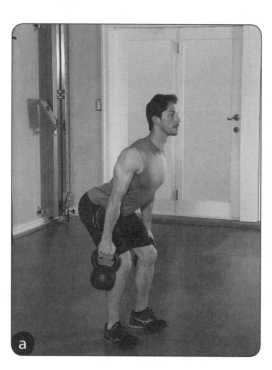
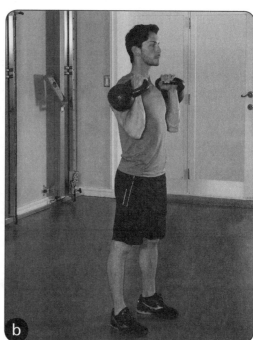

Start

Step 1: Stand with your feet hip-width apart and hold two kettlebells to the outside of your legs.

Step 2: *(a)* Sit back with your hips to stretch your hamstrings and glutes.

Step 3: *(b)* Quickly push your heels into the floor, drive your hips forward, and propel the weights up to the side of your arms by letting the kettlebells rotate to the outside of your forearms.

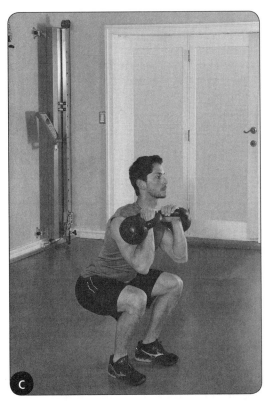

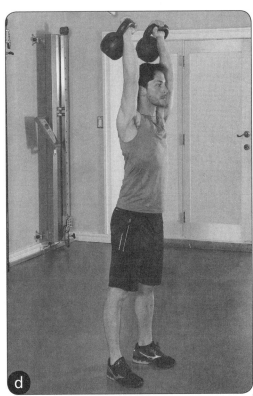

Midpoint

Step 4: *(c)* Catch the kettlebells on the side of your shoulders and arms and then sit back into a deep squat by keeping your weight on your hips and heels. Ensure that your knees stay behind your toes by sitting back with your hips to start the movement.

Step 5: *(d)* After you reach the bottom of your squat, push up hard through your heels and hips. As you are pushing up with your legs you should also be pressing the two kettlebells above your shoulders into a shoulder press (squat press movement). Keep your palms facing away from you throughout the press.

Finish

Step 6: Allow your elbows to bend and return the weight down slowly to your shoulders and then back down beside your legs where you started.

TRAINING TIP

This exercise is really three movements in one. It hits your entire body and definitely gives your metabolism a surge! Start with two lighter kettlebells. As you become more comfortable with the movements you can work your way up safely. Also, remember to keep your chest up throughout the set to protect your back.

DUMBBELL ONE-ARM DEADLIFTS FROM FLOOR

EXERCISE NOTES

- This is the second exercise in the first tri-set of the third workout of the Functional Training Workout.
- Complete this exercise directly after performing kettlebell cleans, front squats, and presses.

Start

Step 1: Place a single heavy dumbbell between your legs on the floor.

Step 2: Standing over the dumbbell, sit back with your hips and keep your weight on your heels.

Step 3: *(a)* Sit into a deep squat and grab the dumbbell with your right hand. Keep your chest up throughout the set.

Midpoint

Step 4: *(b)* With a flat back, forcefully push your heels into the floor and pull the weight up to a standing position. Squeeze your glutes at the top and pull your shoulder blades back.

Finish

Step 5: Squat back down and touch the dumbbell to the floor before performing the next rep. Always pull the weight from the floor by being fully engaged through your legs, back, and core.

Step 6: Repeat all reps on one side and then switch sides.

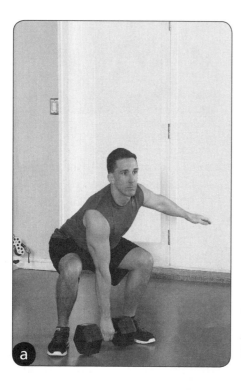 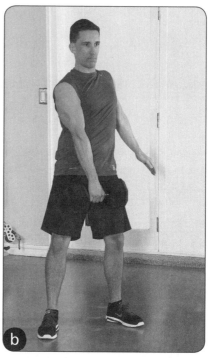

TRAINING TIP

By just using one arm you force your core to work harder to resist any rotation or leaning that your body would like to use to make the lift easier. Keep your torso vertical and core engaged (even at the bottom of the rep).

HANGING KNEE-UPS

EXERCISE NOTES

- This is the third exercise in the third workout of the Functional Training Workout.
- Complete this exercise directly after performing dumbbell one-arm deadlifts from floor.
- Because this is the third exercise in your tri-set, you will rest after completing it.

Start

Step 1: Hold on to a pull-up bar and pull yourself to the top with a supinated chin-up grip or a parallel grip (you can also place your upper arms in the abs straps for support). Hold this position statically throughout the set.

Step 2: *(a)* Engage your core and lift your feet off the floor without swinging.

Midpoint

Step 3: *(b)* Pull your knees up to your elbows using your abs and hip flexors.

Step 4: Slowly lower your legs out at a 45-degree angle to keep the tension on your core.

Finish

Step 5: When your knees reach the point where they are about to lock out, immediately bring them back up to your elbows for your next rep (keeping your core engaged and not pausing at the bottom will help prevent swinging).

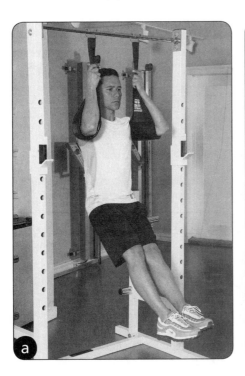
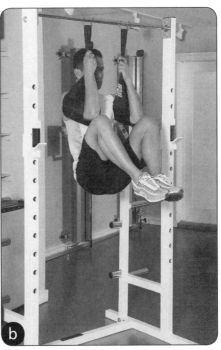

TRAINING TIP

I like this exercise for two reasons: First, it strengthens the core and abs with each rep, and second, it works your back and biceps isometrically as you hold yourself up. By trying to touch your knees to your elbows you get a full range of motion that promotes better abdominal development.

BARBELL SUPINATED INVERTED ROWS

EXERCISE NOTES

- Complete the entire first tri-set three times before moving on to the second group of exercises.
- This is the first exercise in the second tri-set of the third Functional Training Workout.

Start

Step 1: Set up a Smith machine or barbell bench press station so that the barbell is in a fixed and secured position.

Step 2: After you have placed the bar where you want it (the higher the bar is, the easier it will be to complete the exercise), slide under the bar and face up to the ceiling.

Step 3: *(a)* Grip the bar with your palms facing you right in front of your shoulders and stretch your body out under the bar so that your chest lines up directly under it. Make sure that your knees are straight and that your toes point up to the ceiling as well. (I suggest putting your feet up on a box or bench to make this movement more challenging if needed.)

Midpoint

Step 4: *(b)* With your hips lifted and your core and glutes engaged throughout the set, pull your chest up to the bar by squeezing your back muscles and pulling your shoulder blades together.

Finish

Step 5: Allow your body to lower slowly toward the floor without touching, continue to keep tension on your back, and do not allow your shoulders to round forward.

Step 6: Repeat.

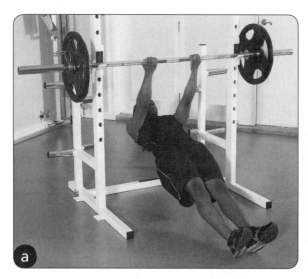
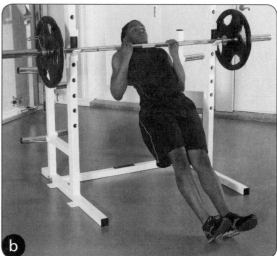

TRAINING TIP

The main point here is to keep your entire body stiff in an upside-down plank position and your core and glutes engaged (don't let your hips sag down toward the floor) so that your back muscles can do their job of pulling your chest up to the bar. Also, focus more on squeezing your shoulder blades together and less on using your arms to pull yourself up.

BARBELL SHOULDER-LOADED WALKING LUNGES

EXERCISE NOTES

- This is the second exercise in the second tri-set of the third workout of the Functional Training Workout.
- Complete this exercise directly after performing barbell supinated inverted rows.

Start

Step 1: *(a)* Step under a squat rack and place a barbell on your trapezius muscles. Hold each side of the barbell beside your shoulders throughout the set to balance the weight.

Step 2: Pull your shoulder blades back and keep them retracted for the remainder of the set.

Step 3: Move away from the squat rack and then step forward with one leg, keeping your weight on the heel of that foot.

Midpoint

Step 4: *(b)* Sit into the hip of the front leg as you lower your back knee into a lunge.

Step 5: Continue to keep the weight on your front hip and heel as you push up through them to propel you back to the top.

Finish

Step 6: Step forward with the back leg as you come to the top of your stance.

Step 7: Repeat by alternating sides.

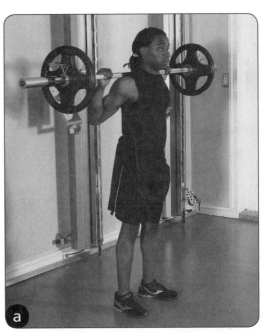

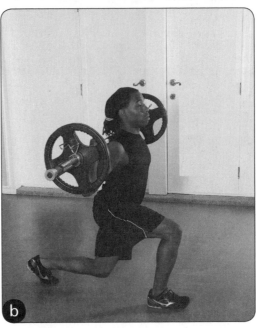

TRAINING TIP

It's important to take a step large enough that you can sit into your front hip and heel without allowing your front knee to go over your toes. Also, if you don't have enough space to do walking lunges, you can keep everything else the same and just substitute the walking movement with backward or forward lunges in place.

KETTLEBELL TWO-ARM SWINGS

EXERCISE NOTES

- This is the third exercise in the second tri-set of the third workout in the Functional Training Workout.
- Complete this exercise directly after performing barbell shoulder-loaded walking lunges.
- Because this is the third exercise in the tri-set, you will rest before repeating.

Start

Step 1: Hold a kettlebell (or dumbbell) between your legs by gripping the handle with both hands.

Step 2: Keep your spine neutral while sitting back with your hips so that you can feel your hamstrings and glutes stretch.

Step 3: (a) Pretend as if you're passing the kettlebell through your legs behind you as you stretch back with your hips.

Midpoint

Step 4: (b) Drive forward and up with your hips to propel yourself to a standing position and allow the kettlebell to swing up and through your legs. The kettlebell should swing to about chest height for our purposes.

Finish

Step 5: Allow the kettlebell to swing down between your legs. Go immediately into your next repetition.

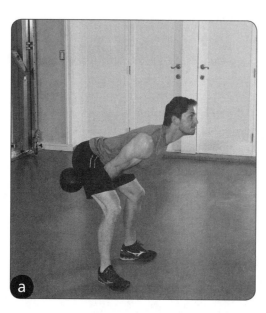
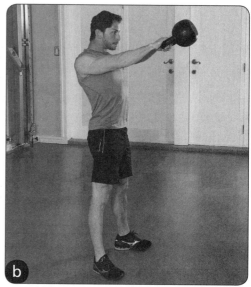

TRAINING TIP

With this exercise we're looking to generate a lot of power, so use a kettlebell that is heavy enough so that you have to thrust your hips forward to get the weight moving up. Although you can hold a dumbbell vertically with both hands on the handle, it is best to do this exercise with a kettlebell. Also, make sure not to swing the weight with your arms but rather use your hips to generate enough power to swing the weight up to about chest height.

CHAPTER 12

Upper-Body Blast Workout

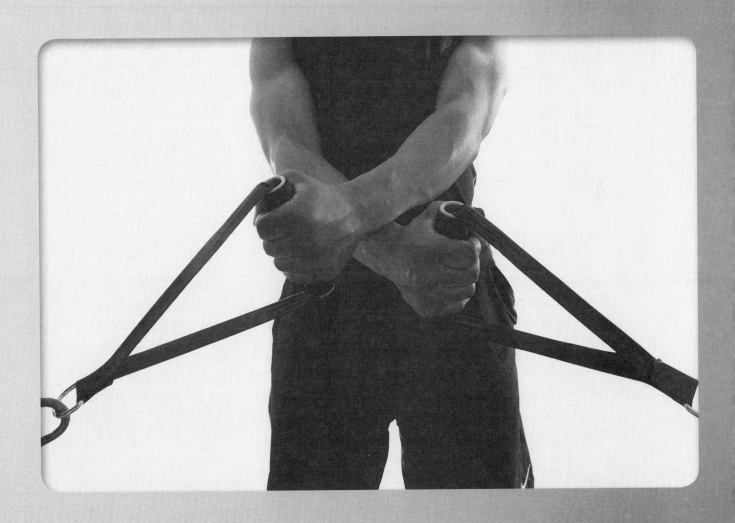

As a guy, you can't deny the fact that training your upper body is just plain fun. Who doesn't like pumping up their arms and chest? And I haven't met a man yet who says that his arms and shoulders are just too big.

Now besides the fact that working out should be fun, there is a lot of merit to training your arms (as long as it doesn't become excessive or the focus of your workouts). By strengthening the muscles that attach to your wrist, elbow, and shoulder joints, you are helping to keep those potentially vulnerable spots strong and stable when performing some of your main strength and power lifts.

For example, you need strong shoulders and triceps to hit your max weights on a bench press, and your biceps and forearms need to be strong enough to complement your back on vertical pulls and horizontals rows.

Having said that, you should be careful when training the upper body so as not to neglect the larger muscle groups. We also want to make sure that we don't do any excessive, repetitive-motion movements that could put your elbow joints at risk for injury.

Having considered all these key elements, I've created for you the ultimate exercise program for the upper body. I've included not only the chest, back, and shoulder exercises that you'll need in your program to keep those muscles big and strong but also a few leg-based movements to increase natural testosterone and growth hormone levels to stimulate new growth. This assortment of exercises will make your program extremely well rounded, so you won't be missing out on anything. You're going to be safely working your arms by attacking your biceps, triceps, shoulders, and forearms from multiple angles and by using varied repetition schemes.

Another important tip when working your arms during a single-joint movement like a biceps curl or triceps press-down in which only the elbow joint is actively working is not to use so much weight that you can't do eight repetitions. I believe that anything less than that number poses too much risk for too little reward. Remember, if you get injured you're out of the game, so it doesn't make any sense to train at or near your breaking point when it comes to a single-joint exercise.

Also, keep in mind that when you're doing a biceps or triceps single-joint exercise you are using your elbow as the fulcrum and your forearm as the lever. What I mean by this is that for the most part your upper arm from your elbow to your shoulder should stay in a fairly fixed position while just your forearm does the moving during the exercise.

By using that method you will create a greater length–tension relationship and allow your biceps or triceps to get a greater training effect. You may need to use a little less weight than you're used to at first, but nonetheless you'll get better results because of the greater stress placed on the muscles that you are targeting. It's a great training technique that you should use to your advantage!

Lastly, I know you're going to love the Upper-Body Blast training program (how could you not!), and I hope you enjoy the gains that you make over the next four to six weeks using it. Make sure to use table 12.1 and tables 12.2 and 12.3 on page 220 as a basis to track your workouts. Now let's get into the top 10 tips I want you to remember in the Upper-Body Blast.

Top 10 Tips and Benefits of the Upper-Body Blast:

1. Sometimes you just need a break from the grind, and the Upper-Body Blast routine will be an enjoyable return to your college training days.

2. This unique program will help you develop bigger and stronger shoulders, triceps, biceps, and forearms while not neglecting your other main muscle groups, including your legs.

3. To keep your joints safe and to maximize your results, I've designed the program to include varied repetition schemes and multiple-angle movements.

4. The Upper-Body Blast was designed in a way to burn body fat so that you don't miss out on any of the metabolic effects of the other workouts.

5. Remember to focus on using your elbow as the fulcrum and your forearm as the lever during each biceps curl or triceps extension.

6. You're going to be amazed how much your core is worked even though you aren't doing any standard crunches or abs exercises.

7. If a movement is brand new to you, be sure to ease into it with a lighter weight until you master the form.

8. Keep in mind that great-looking, well-defined arms are more than just a nice way to fill out your T-shirts. They function as secondary muscle groups in all your major compound lifts.

9. After four to six weeks of consistent training with the Upper-Body Blast routine, you will notice powerful strength and mass increases in the overall look and function of your upper-body muscles.

10. The Upper-Body Blast is a fantastic program that you can add into your training regimen once a year to spice up your old routine or work on any neglected smaller groups!

Table 12.1 Upper-Body Blast Workout, Workout Chart 1

Exercise	Sets	Reps	Tempo	Week 1	Week 2	Week 3	Week 4	Week 5	Week 6
W1. Jumping jacks	1	30 s	1-0-1-0	Weights					
W2. Backward lunge press-outs	1	20	2-0-1-0						
W3. Medicine ball slams	1	15	1-0-1-0						
(Once warm-up exercises are completed, begin strength training.)									
1A. Kettlebell alternating shoulder presses	3	16	2-0-1-0						
1B. Chin-ups	3	8	2-0-1-0						
(Rest 2–3 minutes and repeat exercises 1A and 1B.)									
2A. Dumbbell deadlifts to cheat hammer curls	4	8	3-0-1-1						
2B. Dips	4	8	2-0-1-1						
(Rest 2–3 minutes and repeat exercises 2A and 2B.)									
3A. Cable criss cross raises	3	10	2-0-1-1						
3B. Cable overhead rope triceps extensions	3	10	2-0-1-1						
(Rest 2–3 minutes and repeat exercises 3A and 3B.)									

Table 12.2   Upper-Body Blast Workout, Workout Chart 2

Exercise	Sets	Reps	Tempo	Week 1	Week 2	Week 3	Week 4	Week 5	Week 6
W1. Jumping jacks	1	20	1-0-1-1			Weights			
W2. Backward lunge press-outs	1	20	2-0-1-0						
W3. Medicine ball slams	1	15	1-0-1-0						
(Once warm-up exercises are completed, begin strength training.)									
1A. Medicine ball push-ups	3	AMAP	2-0-1-0						
1B. Cable one-arm horizontal rows	3	2 × 12-10	2-0-1-0						
1C. Bench leg lifts to hip thrusts	3	AMAP	3-0-1-0						
(Rest 2–3 minutes and repeat exercises 1A, 1B, and 1C.)									
2A. Dumbbell squat to standing reverse flys	3	AMAP (10-15)	2-0-1-1						
2B. Cable supinated triceps press-downs	3	12-10	2-0-1-1						
2C. Cable supinated wide-grip biceps curls	3	8-10	2-0-1-1						
(Rest 2–3 minutes and repeat exercises 2A, 2B, and 2C.)									

Table 12.3   Upper-Body Blast Workout, Workout Chart 3

Exercise	Sets	Reps	Tempo	Week 1	Week 2	Week 3	Week 4	Week 5	Week 6
W1. Jumping jacks	1	20	1-0-1-1			Weights			
W2. Backward lunge press-outs	1	20	2-0-1-0						
W3. Medicine ball slams	1	15	1-0-1-0						
(Once warm-up exercises are completed, begin strength training.)									
1A. Barbell push presses	3	15	1-0-1-0						
1B. Dumbbell shrugs	3	15	2-0-1-1						
1C. Cable close-grip triceps press-downs	3	15	2-0-1-1						
1D. Dumbbell Zottman curls	3	15	2-0-1-1						
1E. Kettlebell double swings	3	15	1-0-1-0						
(Rest 2–3 minutes and repeat exercises 1A, 1B, 1C, 1D, and 1E.)									

JUMPING JACKS

EXERCISE NOTES

Complete the dynamic warm-up exercises first before performing all three weight workouts in the Upper-Body Blast Workout.

Start

Step 1: *(a)* Stand with your feet hip-width apart and your hands by your sides.

Step 2: Tighten your core and shift your weight onto the balls of your feet.

Midpoint

Step 3: *(b)* Quickly jump out with one leg to each side, raise your arms overhead at the same time, and land on the balls of your feet.

Step 4: Without resting jump both feet back together while lowering your arms to your sides.

Finish

Step 5: Repeat this motion by rapidly jumping in and out and raising your arms overhead for 30 to 60 seconds.

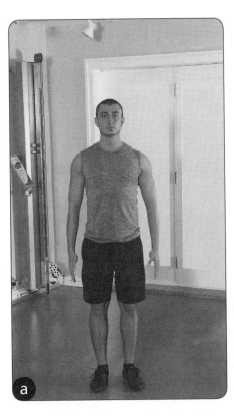 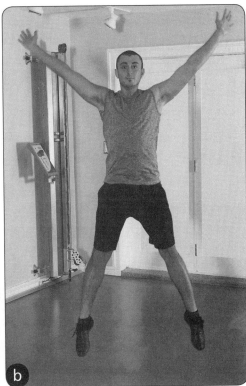

TRAINING TIP

To get the most out of this exercise, be sure to raise both arms all the way overhead to feel the stretch. Also, concentrate on landing softly and absorbing the impact so that your joints stay safe.

BACKWARD LUNGE PRESS-OUTS

EXERCISE NOTES

- Complete the dynamic warm-up exercises first before performing all three weight workouts in the Upper-Body Blast Workout.
- Complete this exercise directly after performing jumping jacks.

Start

Step 1: *(a)* Stand with your feet shoulder-width apart and hold a medicine ball in front of your chest.

Step 2: Step backward with your left leg and land on the ball of that foot.

Midpoint

Step 3: *(b)* Allow your back (left) knee to bend toward the floor but stop it before it touches the ground. At the same time press the medicine ball straight out in front of your chest without leaning forward with your upper body.

Step 4: Allow the weight moving out in front of you to help you sit farther back into your hips.

Finish

Step 5: Bring the medicine ball back into your chest and step forward with your left leg so that you are back in the starting position.

Step 6: Alternate sides and complete the same technique with your right leg.

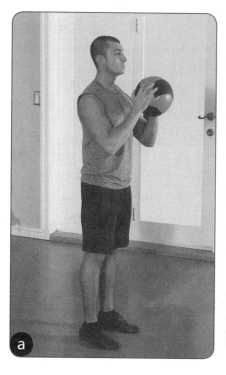
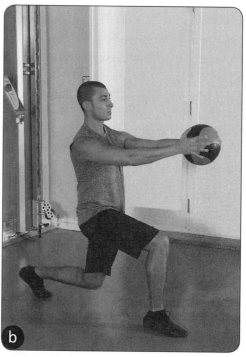

TRAINING TIP

Work on maintaining your balance and posture while trying not to let your back heel touch the floor during your lunge. Also, make sure not to let your front knee go over your toes.

MEDICINE BALL SLAMS

EXERCISE NOTES

- Complete the dynamic warm-up exercises first before performing all three weight workouts in the Upper-Body Blast Workout.
- Complete this exercise directly after performing backward lunge press-outs.

Start

Step 1: Stand with your feet about shoulder-width apart and hold a medicine ball with both hands.

Step 2: *(a)* Raise the medicine ball overhead.

Midpoint

Step 3: *(b)* Quickly flex your core, sit back with your hips, and exhale while slamming the ball from overhead onto the mat between your feet by rapidly bringing both arms down and over your body. (Do not let go of the medicine ball at any time; hold on tight so that it doesn't bounce back up at you!)

Finish

Step 4: Stand back up to the starting position and raise the medicine ball back up overhead.

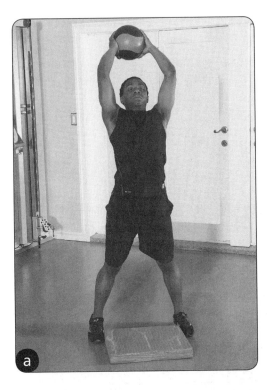
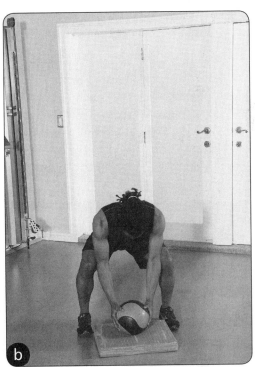

TRAINING TIP

Medicine ball slams are a great way to work your abs and core almost as if you are performing a crunch. The difference is that this exercise is far more functional and is great for developing a lean, mean, and functionally fit midsection. Don't be afraid to slam the ball hard into the floor (use a mat if you're worried about the noise or impact on the floor).

KETTLEBELL ALTERNATING SHOULDER PRESSES

EXERCISE NOTES

- Complete the dynamic warm-up exercises first.
- This is the first exercise in the first workout of the Upper-Body Blast Workout.

Start

Step 1: Stand with your feet shoulder-width apart and hold a pair of kettlebells by your sides.

Step 2: Keep your knees bent and your core engaged throughout the set.

Step 3: *(a)* Lift both kettlebells so that they face away from your shoulders and your palms face your chest and shoulders.

Midpoint

Step 4: *(b)* Press one kettlebell directly overhead by rotating your arm so that the kettlebell faces away from your body but remains right above your shoulder. Do not arch your back while pressing overhead.

Finish

Step 5: Slowly decelerate the weight back to the starting position with your palm facing your chest and shoulder.

Step 6: Maintain form and alternate repetitions.

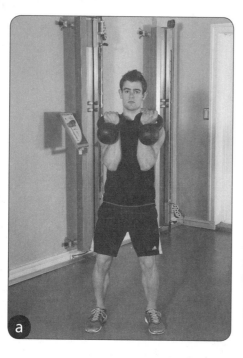 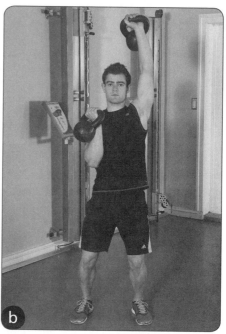

TRAINING TIP

The great thing about this shoulder press is that you're increasing the range of motion in your shoulder capsule while improving overall joint stability throughout the movement. Remember always to engage your abs and core and maintain proper posture. Also, if you do not have kettlebells you can substitute dumbbells for the same movement.

CHIN-UPS

EXERCISE NOTES

- This is the second exercise in the Upper-Body Blast Workout.
- Complete this exercise directly after performing kettlebell alternating shoulder presses.
- Because this is the second exercise in your superset, you will rest after completing it.

Start

Step 1: *(a)* Grip a straight pull-up (chin-up) bar with your hands facing you and lined up directly in front of your shoulders.

Step 2: Engage your core to prevent your body from swinging and then lift your legs off the floor. Crossing your legs can help with stability.

Midpoint

Step 3: *(b)* Use your back muscles and biceps to pull yourself up so that your chest comes up to the bar.

Finish

Step 4: Slowly lower yourself to the point right before your elbows are about to lock out.

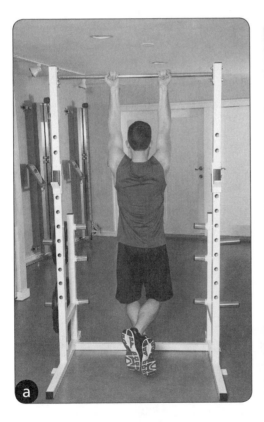
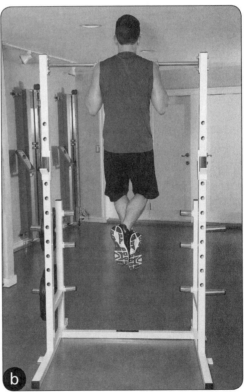

TRAINING TIP

Fight the urge to swing or allow your elbows to lock at the bottom. Keep constant tension on your back and biceps muscles. If you can complete more repetitions than what is recommended, hold a dumbbell between your feet or wear a weighted vest or belt to make the exercise more challenging.

DUMBBELL DEADLIFTS TO CHEAT HAMMER CURLS

EXERCISE NOTES

- Complete the entire first superset three or four times before moving on to the second group of exercises.
- This is the first exercise in the second superset of the Upper-Body Blast Workout.

Start

Step 1: Grab a pair of dumbbells and hold them by your sides.

Step 2: Lift your chest up and retract your shoulder blades.

Step 3: Keeping your core engaged, sit back with your hips while maintaining good posture and keeping your weight on your heels.

Midpoint

Step 4: *(a)* Slowly sit back with your hips as deep as you can into a squat position so that your legs are approximately parallel to the floor. (Make sure to stop before your hips and lower back round out.)

Finish

Step 5: *(b)* Drive through your heels, pull your chest up while exhaling, and push your body back to a standing position. As you are standing back up to the starting position, curl the dumbbells up while keeping a parallel or neutral grip.

Step 6: Allow the dumbbells to uncurl slowly back down toward your sides and then repeat the technique for the desired number of reps.

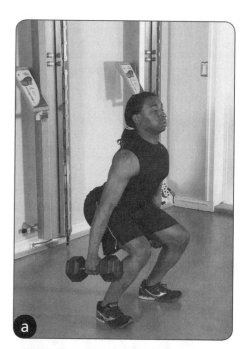

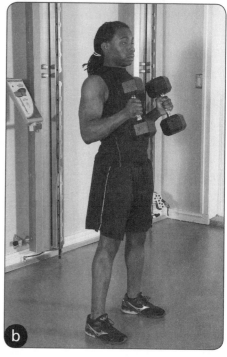

TRAINING TIP

Remember to use all the same tips of keeping a neutral spine and sitting back into your hips while keeping your chest up when you complete the deadlift. In this move, however, you want to use your upward momentum as you begin to stand back up from the bottom of your deadlift to swing the dumbbells up into a curl. Keep in mind that the weights are going to be heavier than you would normally curl with, so you will need a slight controlled swing to get them up to the top. From that point you will uncurl them and get the benefit from the slow negative descent.

DIPS

EXERCISE NOTES

- This is the second exercise in the second superset of the first workout of the Upper-Body Blast Workout.
- Complete this exercise directly after performing dumbbell deadlifts to cheat hammer curls.
- Because this is the second exercise in your superset, you will rest after completing it.

Start

Step 1: Using parallel bar dip handles, grip both sides and tilt your chest slightly forward.

Step 2: *(a)* Hold yourself up in the air and lift your legs off the ground.

Step 3: Keeping your elbows in alignment with your shoulders (do not allow them to flare out), slowly lower yourself down.

Midpoint

Step 4: *(b)* Stop when your biceps are parallel to the ground or just above that point if you are feeling unstable or tight through your shoulders.

Finish

Step 5: Squeeze your triceps while straightening your elbows and push yourself to the starting position.

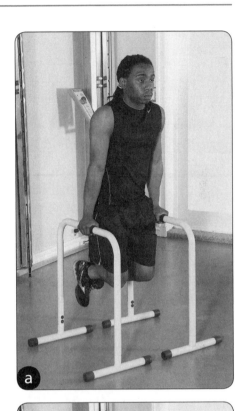

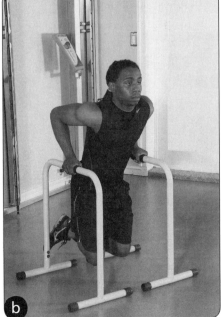

TRAINING TIP

I'm a huge fan of dips for triceps, shoulder, and chest development, but you must be careful to keep the tension on those muscles all the way through the movement. Be sure not to stretch too deep and cause too much shoulder flexion. Also, if you can complete more repetitions than what is recommended, I suggest holding a dumbbell between your feet or wearing a weighted vest or belt to make the exercise more challenging.

CABLE CRISS CROSS RAISES

EXERCISE NOTES

- Complete the first two supersets before moving on to this last superset.
- This is the first exercise in the third superset of the Upper-Body Blast Workout.

Start

Step 1: Attach two handles at the bottom pulleys of two cable arms or towers.

Step 2: *(a)* Grab both handles by reaching across with your right hand to grab the left handle and with your left hand to grab the right handle. Stand up to your starting position with your feet about shoulder-width apart (no wider). The cables should now be crisscrossed in front of your hips to form an X.

Step 3: Tighten your core before you raise the handles so that you do not arch your back.

Midpoint

Step 4: *(b)* Keeping your wrists straight and having only a 10-degree bend in your elbows, raise both handles up to the sides of your body. You finish at the top with your shoulders, elbows, and wrists all on the same plane and forming a straight line.

Finish

Step 5: After briefly pausing at the top, slowly decelerate your arms down without allowing your core to disengage or your shoulders to lose tension. Stop at the point where the handles reach the outsides of your hips.

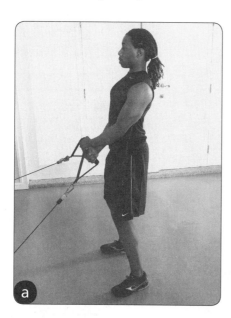
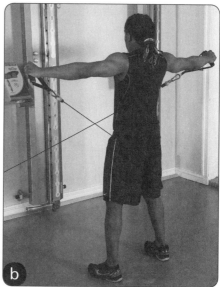

TRAINING TIP

A lot of guys have a difficult time completing a lateral raise by focusing only on the shoulder muscles, so I suggest pretending that you are pouring a pitcher of your favorite beverage out as you raise the weights with slightly bent elbows. By the time you reach the top, you should have your thumbs pointed slightly down to the floor and your elbows just above your hands.

CABLE OVERHEAD ROPE TRICEPS EXTENSIONS

EXERCISE NOTES

- This is the second exercise in third superset of the first workout of the Upper-Body Blast Workout.
- Complete this exercise directly after performing cable criss cross raises.
- Because this is the second exercise in your superset, you will rest after completing it.

Start

Step 1: Attach a rope to the top pulley of a cable machine.

Step 2: Grab both ends of the rope (right above the knobs) and then rotate your entire body so that it faces away from the cable machine.

Step 3: Engage your core and step a few feet (a meter or so) away from the machine. Maintain a staggered stance with one foot in front of the other and your upper body leaning slightly forward but do not round your lower back. Look straight ahead throughout the set.

Midpoint

Step 4: *(a)* At this point your elbows should be bent at about right angles and fixed around your temples. *(b)* Now extend just your forearms straight out in front of you, spreading the ends of the rope out so that they come out as wide as your shoulders.

Finish

Step 5: After briefly squeezing your triceps at full extension slowly bend at the elbows (keeping them in tight) and allow your forearms to move back to the starting position while stretching your triceps.

TRAINING TIP

I like this exercise not only for the great triceps building effect that it has but also for the way that it works your core. Remember not to move the upper arm much; use the forearms to do the moving. Additionally, it's the triceps that flex on the way out and stretch on the way back, so focus on how they feel throughout the set.

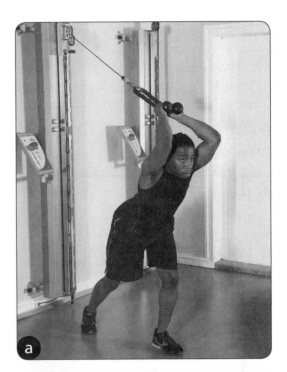
a

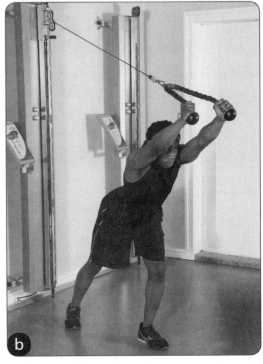
b

MEDICINE BALL PUSH-UPS

EXERCISE NOTES

- Complete the dynamic warm-up exercises first.
- This is the first exercise in the second workout of the Upper-Body Blast Workout.

Start

Step 1: *(a)* Place a medicine ball on the floor beneath your chest. Hold the medicine ball with both hands so that your palms face each other and get up on the balls of your feet in a push-up position. Your feet should be together.

Step 2: *(b)* Decelerate your chest down toward the ball into a push-up without letting your hips sag. Be sure to keep your elbows in tight to your sides as you come down toward the ball.

Midpoint

Step 3: As you push back up to the top, do not allow your hips to drop down or your elbows to flare out. Maintain a tight core throughout the set.

Finish

Step 4: After briefly pausing at the top, slowly lower yourself down into your next medicine ball push-up.

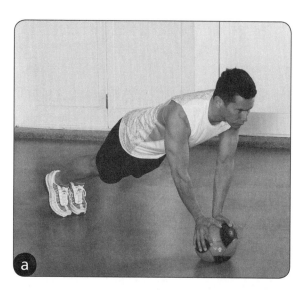
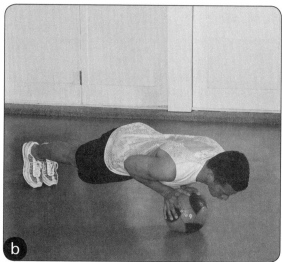

TRAINING TIP

Remember not to drop your hips as you lower yourself down. Also, if you're having a difficult time with this exercise, you can start by doing diamond push-ups without the ball or by not getting too deep into your eccentric lowering phase. In time you'll be able to get deeper into each push-up without resting at the bottom. My last point is to keep your triceps in tight to your body so that you protect your joints and keep the tension where it should be emphasized.

CABLE ONE-ARM HORIZONTAL ROWS

EXERCISE NOTES

- This is the second exercise in the Upper-Body Blast Workout.
- Complete this exercise directly after performing medicine ball push-ups.

Start

Step 1: With your left hand grab a single cable attached at shoulder height.

Step 2: *(a)* Step backward with your left leg into a staggered stance so that the cable is under tension at all times.

Step 3: Point your palm toward the floor and keep your wrist, elbow, and shoulder on the same plane.

Midpoint

Step 4: *(b)* Pull the cable toward your left shoulder by forcefully squeezing the muscles on the left side of your back while stretching the muscles of your left pectorals. Exhale while pulling in.

Finish

Step 5: Slowly decelerate the weight back to the starting position while feeling your back and shoulder muscles stretch. Keep your core engaged and your legs rooted into the ground so that you do not allow your body to be pulled forward toward the weight stack. Breathe in as the weight returns to its starting position.

Step 6: Repeat on the left side and then move on to the right.

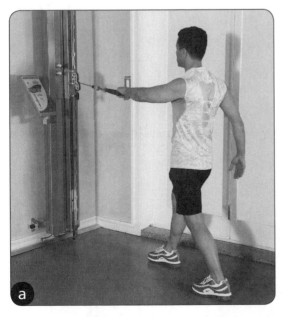
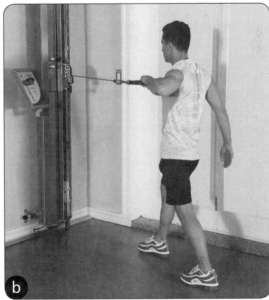

TRAINING TIP

Use your obliques, core, and legs to stabilize your entire body while looking at the cable attachment in front of you throughout the set. Feel the muscles in your back contracting as you pull the handle away from the cable machine.

BENCH LEG LIFTS TO HIP THRUSTS

EXERCISE NOTES

- This is the third exercise in the Upper-Body Blast Workout.
- Complete this exercise directly after performing cable one-arm horizontal rows.
- Because this is the third exercise in your tri-set, you will rest after completing it.

Start

Step 1: Lie on your back on a bench with your hips half on and half off the edge of the bench.

Step 2: Hold on to the bench beside your head.

Step 3: Begin by stretching your legs out straight and then lifting them up in a leg lift movement until your feet come right above your hips (keep your knees straight throughout the set).

Midpoint

Step 4: *(a)* Push your upper back deeper into the bench and thrust your hips up in the air with your legs moving toward the ceiling.

Step 5: Slowly lower your hips back down to the bench.

Finish

Step 6: *(b)* Finally, lower your legs back down toward the floor. Just before your legs touch, lift them back up and repeat.

TRAINING TIP

This exercise has dozens of variations. For example, to make the movement easier, you can bend your knees, do a reverse crunch with your legs pulling into your hips, and then thrust up. To make it more difficult, you could leg lift up, hip thrust, and then instead of lowering your hips to the bench, immediately go right into the negative of a leg lift toward the floor (often called a dragon flag). I prefer the method that I outlined here because it falls somewhere in the middle and allows you to focus on the two separate movements.

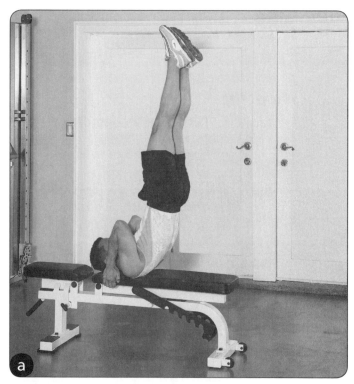

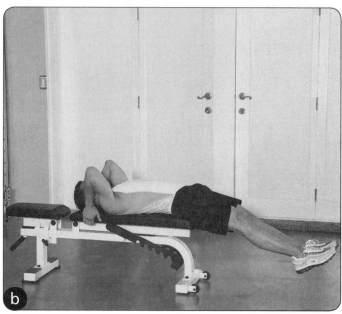

DUMBBELL SQUAT TO STANDING REVERSE FLYS

EXERCISE NOTES

- Complete the entire first tri-set two or three times before moving on to the second group of exercises.
- This is the first exercise in the second tri-set of the Upper-Body Blast Workout.

Start

Step 1: Hold a pair of dumbbells 3 to 4 inches (about 8 to 10 cm) apart in front of your hips.

Step 2: *(a)* Sit back on your hips and heels into a deep squat, hold your chest high, and hold the dumbbells beside your knees.

Midpoint

Step 3: *(b)* As you stand back up to the starting position raise both dumbbells up in the air at a 45-degree angle over your shoulders and have your palms facing away from you. As you get to the top of your movement you should have both arms raised over your shoulders as if you were holding your arms up in victory.

Finish

Step 4: Slowly decelerate the weights back down in front of your body as you squat back down into your next repetition.

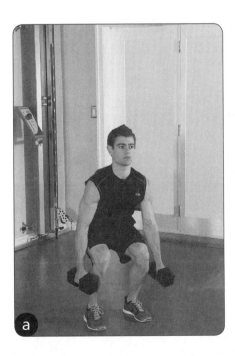
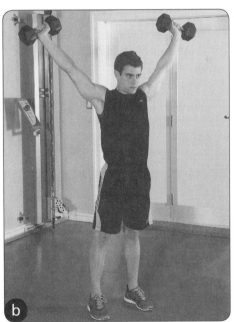

TRAINING TIP

This exercise gets your whole body moving while working on posture and upper-body shoulder strength. Here are a few key tips to remember: (1) Keep a 10-degree bend in your elbows throughout the set; (2) do not arch you back as you raise the weights overhead; (3) squeeze the back of your shoulder blades together as you raise the weights up high in the air.

CABLE SUPINATED TRICEPS PRESS-DOWNS

EXERCISE NOTES

- This is the second exercise in the second tri-set of the Upper-Body Blast Workout.
- Complete this exercise directly after performing dumbbell squat to standing reverse flys.

Start

Step 1: Attach an EZ-bar to the top cable pulley above your head.

Step 2: Using an underhand grip hold the bar toward the ends so that your palms face the ceiling.

Step 3: *(a)* Keep your chest up, engage your core, and place one foot under the bar and one foot behind you in a staggered stance.

Midpoint

Step 4: *(b)* Squeezing your triceps, press the bar down and extend your elbows straight until they cannot go any farther. The bar should end up in front of the forward leg.

Step 5: After pausing for a second at the bottom to squeeze and flex your triceps, slowly allow your elbows to bend and let the bar come back up (do not let your elbows move from your sides during the set).

Finish

Step 6: After your forearms touch your biceps and just before you are about to lose tension on your triceps, press back down again for your next repetition.

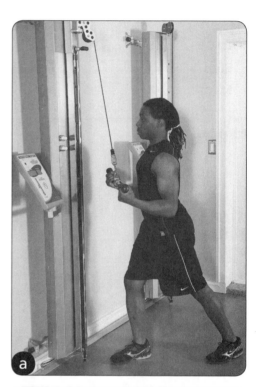

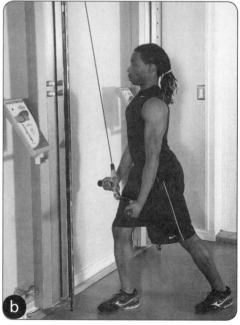

TRAINING TIP

Although you can't press down as much weight using a supinated underhand grip, it is an excellent way to target your triceps from a different angle. By hitting your muscles from multiple attack points, you will develop bigger, stronger muscles and more stable joints.

CABLE SUPINATED WIDE-GRIP BICEPS CURLS

EXERCISE NOTES

- This is the third exercise in the second tri-set of the Upper-Body Blast Workout.
- Complete this exercise directly after performing cable supinated triceps press-downs.
- Because this is the third exercise in your tri-set, you will rest after completing it.

Start

Step 1: Take the cable attachment and EZ-bar that you just used for the triceps press-downs and move the pulley down to the bottom position.

Step 2: Using an underhand grip hold the bar toward the ends using a wide grip so that your palms face the ceiling.

Step 3: *(a)* Keep your chest up, engage your core, and keep both feet about hip- to shoulder-width apart in a parallel stance. Stand up with the bar and let it rest for a moment near your quads.

Midpoint

Step 4: *(b)* Squeezing your biceps lift the bar up toward your chest until your forearms press up against your biceps, stopping the movement. Do not allow your elbows to come forward away from your sides.

Step 5: After pausing for a second at the top to squeeze more blood into your biceps, slowly lower the bar all the way down until your elbows are about to lock out and you lose tension on your biceps.

Finish

Step 6: Do not pause or rest at the bottom; go immediately into your next repetition, keeping constant tension on your biceps.

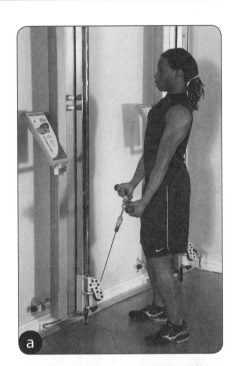

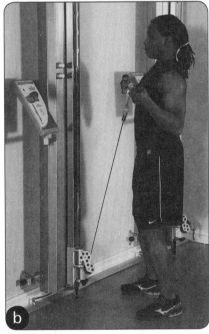

TRAINING TIP

Unlike underhand triceps press-downs this will be one of your strongest biceps curls. You're definitely going to feel "the pump" after completing each set! Just don't make the mistake that many guys do of letting their elbows come up in front of them so that they can rest at the top of each rep. You may not be able to use as much weight by keeping stricter form, but the results will pay off in bigger, stronger arms!

BARBELL PUSH PRESSES

EXERCISE NOTES

- Complete the dynamic warm-up exercises first.
- This is the first exercise in the third workout of the Upper-Body Blast Workout.
- This third workout of the Upper-Body Blast is circuit based, so you will complete all five exercises in a row without resting.
- After you complete all five exercises you can rest for two to three minutes before repeating the entire circuit.

Start

Step 1: Hold a barbell just beyond shoulder-width apart.

Step 2: Place the barbell about 1 inch (2.5 cm) above your shoulders and collarbones.

Step 3: *(a)* Sit back into a quarter squat into your hips and heels while keeping the bar above your chest and shoulders.

Midpoint

Step 4: *(b)* Rapidly stand up straight, driving your feet into the floor and propelling the bar above your head into a shoulder press.

Finish

Step 5: Slowly decelerate the barbell back to the starting position as you move back into your quarter squat.

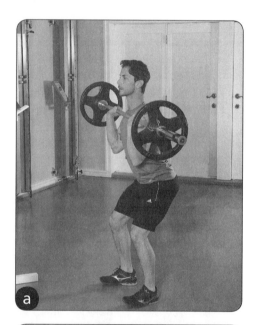

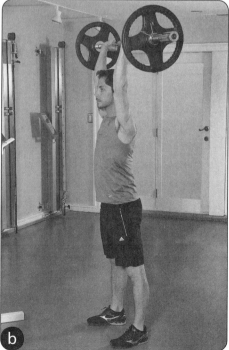

TRAINING TIP

The barbell push press is an excellent way to increase your core, leg, and shoulder strength and power all in one exercise! You can lift a heavier weight than you would typically be able to shoulder press, which also makes it a good way to increase muscle mass and strength.

DUMBBELL SHRUGS

EXERCISE NOTES

- This is the second exercise in the Upper-Body Blast Workout.
- Complete this exercise directly after performing barbell push presses.

Start

Step 1: *(a)* Hold a pair of dumbbells with a tight grip by your sides.

Step 2: Engage your core, do not let your shoulders round forward, and keep your knees slightly bent. Your arms should remain straight throughout the set.

Midpoint

Step 3: *(b)* Look straight ahead and shrug your shoulders up as high as you can toward your ears.

Step 4: Hold and squeeze the upper trapezius muscles at the top.

Finish

Step 5: Slowly lower your shoulders back down until your trapezius muscles fully stretch without you rounding your shoulders forward.

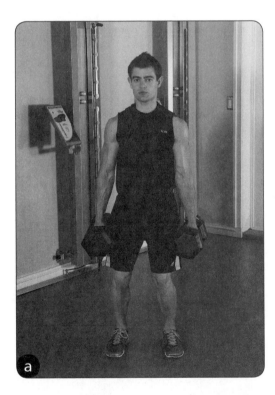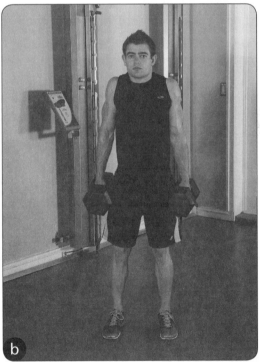

TRAINING TIP

This straightforward exercise allows you to lift the maximum weight possible. The key is to use a full range of motion by trying to touch your shoulders to your ears with each concentric squeeze up with the dumbbells. Although the pull upward with your traps should be fast, your eccentric lowering movement of the bar back to the starting position should be slow.

CABLE CLOSE-GRIP TRICEPS PRESS-DOWNS

EXERCISE NOTES

- This is the third exercise in the third workout of the Upper-Body Blast Workout.
- Complete this exercise directly after performing dumbbell shrugs.

Start

Step 1: Attach a triangle or V-bar to the top cable pulley above your head.

Step 2: Using an overhand grip hold the bar toward the middle so that your palms face the floor.

Step 3: (a) Keep your chest up, engage your core, and place one foot under the bar and one foot behind you in a staggered stance.

Midpoint

Step 4: (b) Squeezing your triceps, press the bar down and extend your elbows straight until they cannot go any farther. The bar should end up in front of the forward leg.

Step 5: After pausing for a second at the bottom to squeeze and flex your triceps, slowly allow your elbows to bend and let the bar come back up (do not let your elbows move from your sides during the set).

Finish

Step 6: After your forearms touch your biceps and just before you are about to lose tension on your triceps, press back down again for your next repetition.

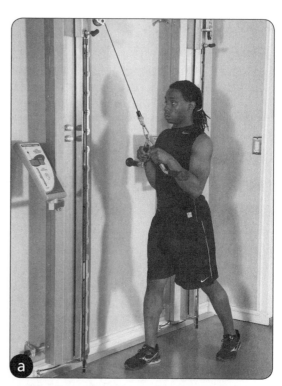

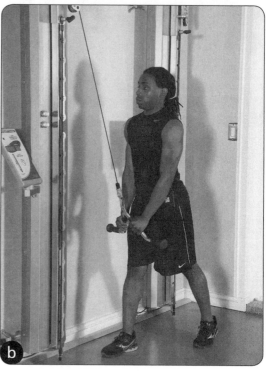

TRAINING TIP

Unlike the underhand triceps press-down, this overhand close-grip press-down allows you to use the maximum weight possible with your triceps. Because you'll be pressing a lot of weight down, make sure to keep your core engaged and do not lean too far over the handle; keep the tension on your triceps the whole time! (If you do not have a V-bar, any attachment will suffice using an overhand close grip.)

DUMBBELL ZOTTMAN CURLS

EXERCISE NOTES

- This is the fourth exercise in the third workout of the Upper-Body Blast Workout.
- Complete this exercise directly after performing cable close-grip triceps press-downs.

Start

Step 1: *(a)* Stand with your feet hip-width apart and hold a pair of dumbbells by your sides.

Step 2: Keep your chest up, shoulder blades retracted, knees bent, and chin parallel to the ground throughout the set.

Step 3: *(b)* Moving just your forearms, rotate both dumbbells as you curl so that your palms face up. Exhale at this point to help produce more force.

Midpoint

Step 4: Forcefully squeeze your biceps without allowing your elbows to pull forward or your shoulder blades to round.

Step 5: *(c)* When you reach the top of your curl, rotate your forearms and wrists so that your palms face the floor.

Finish

Step 6: Slowly lower the weights to your legs, keeping your palms facing down the whole way.

Step 7: Return the weights to your starting position and repeat.

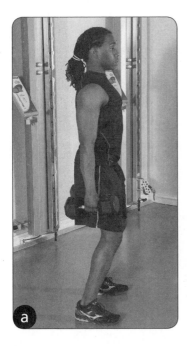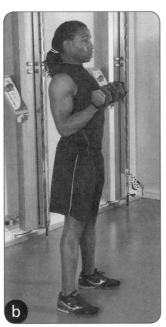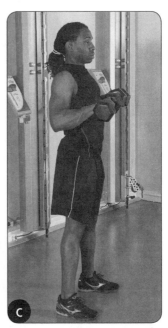

TRAINING TIP

This little known exercise challenges both your biceps and your forearms. Because it is a slightly more complex movement than a traditional dumbbell curl and uses the eccentric motion of a reverse forearm biceps curl, I suggest using a lighter weight to start—you can always go heavier later!

KETTLEBELL DOUBLE SWINGS

EXERCISE NOTES

- Complete this exercise after performing dumbbell Zottman curls.
- This is the fifth exercise in the third workout of the Upper-Body Blast Workout.
- Because this is the final exercise of the circuit, you will rest two or three minutes after completing it before beginning the five-exercise circuit again.

Start

Step 1: Hold two kettlebells (or dumbbells), one in each hand, between your legs.

Step 2: Keep your spine neutral while sitting back with your hips so that you can feel your hamstrings and glutes stretch.

Step 3: *(a)* Pretend that you're passing the kettlebells through your legs behind you as you stretch back with your hips.

Midpoint

Step 4: *(b)* Drive forward and up using your hips to propel yourself to a standing position and allowing both kettlebells to swing up and through your legs. The kettlebells should swing to about chest height for our purposes and should be moving in unison.

Finish

Step 5: Allow both kettlebells to swing down at the same time between your legs. Go immediately into your next repetition.

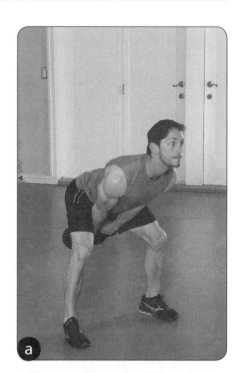

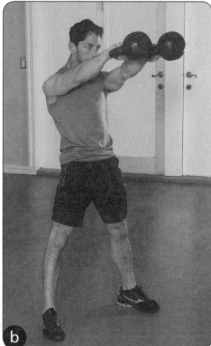

TRAINING TIP

This exercise works your entire body and really pushes your coordination and concentration to a higher level. It takes a significant deal of neuromuscular timing to use the momentum of the kettlebells and the thrusting of your hips to keep the weight moving in sync. After you get the hang of it, you'll feel your muscles screaming and your heart pounding! (Although you can hold dumbbells vertically with both hands, it is best to do this exercise with two kettlebells.)

CHAPTER 13

Hardcore Body-Weight Training Workout

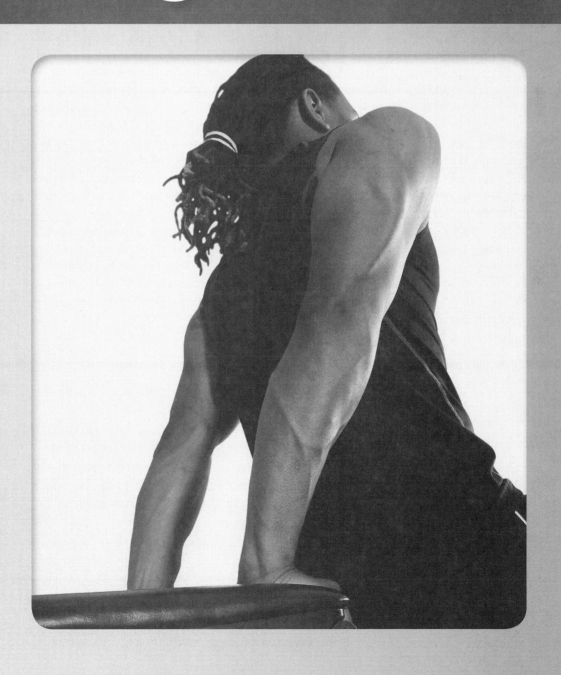

Did you know that mastering your body weight is probably the most important thing you should do before even thinking about touching a weight? It's true. Gaining complete control over your muscles, nervous system, and joint stability is paramount when it comes to staying injury free and developing a strong, athletic-looking body. There simply isn't any substitute for being able to rattle off some advanced push-up maneuvers or a handful of deep one-leg pistol squats.

The issue that I think most guys have with training with just their own body weight is that they think it's going to be too easy. To be honest, for many advanced lifters that's probably the case with most standard body-weight programs. The good news is that the program I developed for you is far from standard.

This Hardcore Body-Weight Training routine will have you burning body fat, feeling the intensity with every rep, and shaking your head wondering how it can be so challenging when it uses no equipment besides your own body.

The truth is that I built this program for my private clients who did not want to miss a workout when they went on vacation or travelled for work. They knew that they might have only 20 minutes to complete a workout in a hotel room, so I had to develop a program that could fit their limited access.

I'm happy to say that the Hardcore Body-Weight Training program has been battle tested and approved by some of my more discriminating clients, so I know that you'll enjoy using it as well. I highly recommend taking this book with you when you travel so that you'll never have an excuse to miss a workout! Make sure to use table 13.1 and tables 13.2 and 13.3 on page 244 as a basis to track your workouts.

One other point is that some of my clients are fathers who aren't able to get out of the house on the weekends to hit the gym for an hour or so. At times like that they can just pull out this chapter and complete a body-weight workout in the basement, in the bedroom, or right in the living room with the kids (kids love these exercises, too).

So whether you're using this program to develop stronger joints, unbreakable connective tissue, denser muscles, a more athletic body, or any other of the hundreds of reasons to master your own body weight, I'm excited for you to try this Hardcore Body-Weight Training program. It is the answer that you've been looking for in terms of getting in a legitimate workout even when you don't have weights at your disposal. Now let's talk about the top 10 tips and benefits that I want you to remember in Hardcore Body-Weight Training.

Top 10 Tips and Benefits of Hardcore Body-Weight Training:

1. Now there's no excuse to miss a workout! You can take this program with you anywhere and complete it with no equipment.

2. This is the perfect program to take on a vacation or a work travel trip during which you may only be able to sneak in a quick workout in your hotel room.

3. The workouts can be done for two sets, which would take approximately 20 minutes to complete, or you can opt for the entire three-set program, which would take 30 to 35 minutes depending on how quickly you move through it.

4. Hardcore Body-Weight Training was designed in a unique way that allows you to train your entire body without creating any imbalances (unlike 99 percent of standard body-weight workouts).

5. Although these workouts involve you using your body weight only, the exercises aren't easy. My suggestion is to start slow and make sure that your form is on point before you move faster or deeper.

6. With most body-weight exercises the way that you make the exercise more challenging is to get deeper into the movement (using a safe range of motion only), add more repetitions, hold each rep longer, or take less rest.

7. Many of my clients use these exercises as games to challenge their friends to see who is truly stronger because each of you is working with his own body weight. Have some fun with the exercises!

8. By mastering all these moves you will find that when you go back to some of the larger compound exercises like the bench press and squat, you are stronger because you have better neuromuscular control and joint and connective tissue strength and stability.

9. After experimenting with this Hardcore Body-Weight Training routine, you will never look at body-weight training the same way again. You may even look forward to using these travel workouts more often!

10. Hardcore Body-Weight Training is the ultimate way to gain athletic power, strength, and control over your entire body. After you master your body weight you will have a deeper appreciation for what you are capable of!

Table 13.1 Hardcore Body-Weight Training Workout, Workout Chart 1

Exercise	Sets	Reps	Tempo	Week 1	Week 2	Week 3	Week 4	Week 5	Week 6
W1. Jumping jacks	1	30 s	1-0-1-0			Weights			
W2. Transverse plane lunges	1	20	2-0-1-0						
W3. Mountain climbers	1	30 s	AFAP*						
(Once warm-up exercises are completed, begin strength training.)									
1A. T-twist push-ups	3	10-20	1-0-1-0						
1B. One-leg pistol squats	3	2 × 8-10	3-0-1-0						
1C. One-leg-up crunches	3	2 × 10-15	2-0-1-1						
(Rest 2–3 minutes and repeat exercises 1A, 1B, and 1C.)									
2A. Side planks with reach under	3	2 × 15	2-0-1-0						
2B. Bulgarian split squats with two-arm raise	3	2 × 15	3-0-1-0						
2C. Alternating supermans	3	20-24	1-0-1-1						
(Rest 2–3 minutes and repeat exercises 2A, 2B, and 2C.)									

*AFAP = As fast as possible.

Table 13.2 Hardcore Body-Weight Training Workout, Workout Chart 2

Exercise	Sets	Reps	Tempo	Week 1	Week 2	Week 3	Week 4	Week 5	Week 6
W1. Jumping jacks	1	30 s	1-0-1-0	Weights					
W2. Transverse plane lunges	1	20	2-0-1-0						
W3. Mountain climbers	1	30 s	AFAP*						
(Once warm-up exercises are completed, begin strength training.)									
1A. Inchworms	3	8-10	3-0-3-0						
1B. Alternating dynamic forward lunges	3	24-30	2-0-1-0						
1C. Chair dips	3	10-15	3-0-1-0						
(Rest 2–3 minutes and repeat exercises 1A, 1B, and 1C.)									
2A. Planks with shoulder abduction	3	24-30	1-0-1-1						
2B. Shin slap V-ups	3	AMAP (10-20)	1-0-1-0						
2C. One-leg dynamic bridging	3	2 × 15	2-0-1-1						
(Rest 2–3 minutes and repeat exercises 2A, 2B, and 2C.)									

*AFAP = As fast as possible.

Table 13.3 Hardcore Body-Weight Training Workout, Workout Chart 3

Exercise	Sets	Reps	Tempo	Week 1	Week 2	Week 3	Week 4	Week 5	Week 6
W1. Jumping jacks	1	30 s	1-0-1-0	Weights					
W2. Transverse plane lunges	1	20	2-0-1-0						
W3. Mountain climbers	1	30 s	AFAP*						
(Once warm-up exercises are completed, begin strength training.)									
1A. Hindu push-ups	3	10	2-0-2-0						
1B. Prisoner deep squats	3	20	2-0-1-0						
1C. Brazilian crunches	3	20-30	1-0-1-0						
1D. One-leg good mornings	3	2 × 12-15	3-0-1-0						
1E. Squat thrusts (burpees)	3	10	AFAP*						
(Rest 2–3 minutes and repeat exercises 1A, 1B, 1C, 1D, and 1E.)									

*AFAP = As fast as possible.

JUMPING JACKS

EXERCISE NOTES

Complete the dynamic warm-up exercises first before performing all three weight workouts in Hardcore Body-Weight Training Workout.

Start

Step 1: *(a)* Stand with your feet slightly apart and your hands by your sides.

Step 2: Tighten your core and shift your weight onto the balls of your feet.

Midpoint

Step 3: *(b)* Quickly jump out with one leg to each side, raise your arms overhead at the same time, and land on the balls of your feet.

Step 4: Without resting jump both feet back together while lowering your arms to your sides.

Finish

Step 5: Repeat this motion by rapidly jumping in and out and raising your arms overhead for 30 to 60 seconds.

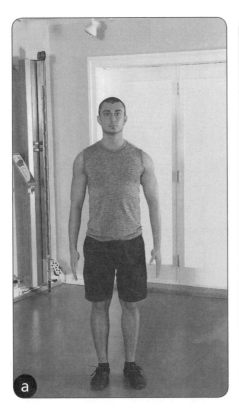
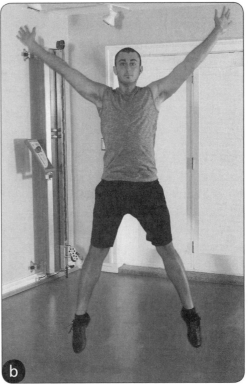

TRAINING TIP

To get the most out of this exercise, be sure to raise both arms all the way overhead to feel the stretch. Also, concentrate on landing softly and absorbing the impact so that your joints stay safe.

TRANSVERSE PLANE LUNGES

EXERCISE NOTES

- Complete the dynamic warm-up exercises first before performing all three weight workouts in Hardcore Body-Weight Training Workout.
- Complete this exercise directly after performing jumping jacks.

Start

Step 1: *(a)* Stand with your feet together.

Step 2: Think of yourself as standing on the twelve o'clock position on a clock. *(b)* Standing on twelve o'clock take a big step to your right so that you land at the three o'clock position on the clock. (Your right foot will now be turned out at a right angle facing three o'clock and perpendicular to your left leg, which remains at twelve o'clock.)

Midpoint

Step 3: Absorb the landing of your right foot by keeping the weight back into your heel and decelerating into your right hip.

Step 4: Do not allow your right knee to go over the toes of your right foot; keep sitting back into your hips. Also, straighten your left leg fully and feel the stretch on the inner thigh of that leg.

Finish

Step 5: Push through your right hip and heel and accelerate back to the starting position, bringing both feet together and standing up straight so that both feet are standing on twelve o'clock and facing forward.

Step 6: Repeat the same technique on the opposite side by lunging with your left leg onto the nine o'clock position. Your left leg will now be bent, and your right leg will be straight.

TRAINING TIP

Although this exercise works to open up your hips by using the rotational plane of motion, make sure that you do not overtwist your upper torso, which should remain square with your hips throughout the set.

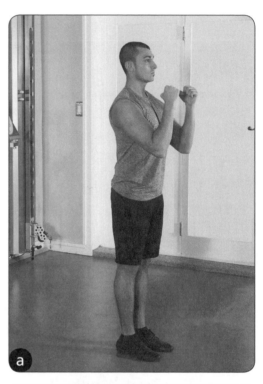

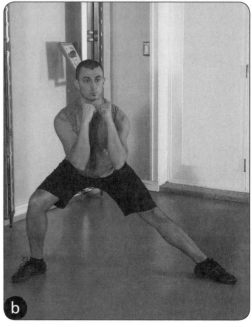

MOUNTAIN CLIMBERS

EXERCISE NOTES

- Complete the dynamic warm-up exercises first before performing all three weight workouts in Hardcore Body-Weight Training Workout.
- Complete this exercise directly after performing transverse plane lunges.

Start

Step 1: Place both hands below your shoulders as you get into a push-up position on the floor.

Step 2: Align the balls of your feet under your ankles so that only your feet and hands are in contact with the ground.

Step 3: Tighten your core.

Midpoint

Step 4: *(a)* Pull one leg off the floor and draw it into your belly while keeping the other leg anchored on the ground.

Step 5: *(b)* Quickly place the leg in the air back on the floor and pull the other leg off the floor and into your belly.

Finish

Step 6: Repeat this motion by rapidly bringing one leg in while the other one works to balance you along with your upper body. Move as quickly as you can for 30 to 60 seconds.

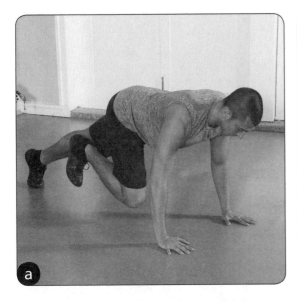
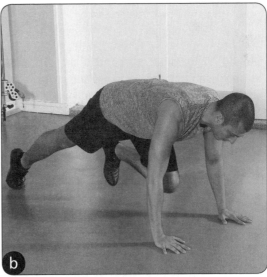

TRAINING TIP

To stay balanced on only three points, remember to keep your core engaged. Also, to reduce stress on your knee joint, do not allow the front foot to touch the floor when you pull it into your belly.

T-TWIST PUSH-UPS

EXERCISE NOTES

- Complete the dynamic warm-up exercises first.
- This is the first exercise in the first workout of Hardcore Body-Weight Training Workout.

Start

Step 1: *(a)* Place both hands on the floor just past your shoulders and get up on the balls of your feet in a push-up position. Your feet should be about hip-width apart.

Step 2: *(b)* Decelerate your chest down toward the floor into a push-up without letting your hips sag.

Midpoint

Step 3: *(c)* As you push back up to the top, allow your entire body to rotate to the right so that your feet domino onto the outside of your left foot and the inside of your right foot. Your outside right arm should rise up above your shoulder to form a straight line with the left arm that is supporting you on the bottom. Your entire body should form a T.

Finish

Step 4: After briefly pausing at the top, slowly decelerate the side of your body that is in the air down to the floor and back into a push-up position. Allow your feet to return to the balls of your feet as well.

Step 5: Complete another push-up and alternate sides, this time twisting to your left. Continue alternating for the desired number of reps.

TRAINING TIP

Remember not to drop your hips as you open up to one side. Doing so will disengage your obliques and entire core and may cause you to lose balance. Take your time and work on becoming comfortable with the movement.

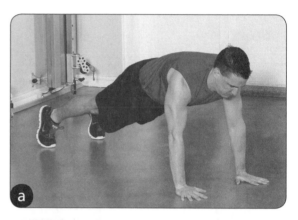

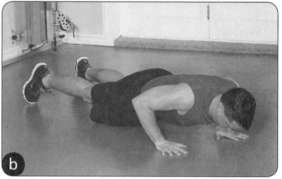

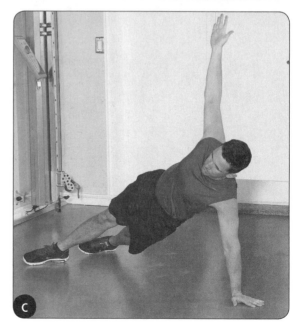

ONE-LEG PISTOL SQUATS

EXERCISE NOTES

- This is the second exercise in Hardcore Body-Weight Training Workout.
- Complete this exercise directly after performing T-twist push-ups.

Start

Step 1: Place a low chair or box behind you if possible (not needed for advanced levels).

Step 2: *(a)* Lift your left leg up in the air and hold it straight out in front of your body.

Step 3: Sit back with your hips and place the weight onto your right heel as you begin to squat down.

Midpoint

Step 4: *(b)* Get as deep as you can into a squat while keeping your core engaged and your arms up in front of your chest for balance.

Finish

Step 5: Push up through your right heel and hips to the standing position. Do not let your left leg touch the floor throughout the set if possible.

Step 6: Repeat all reps on your right side and then move on to the left leg.

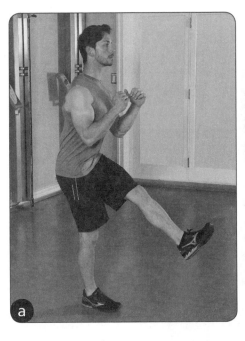 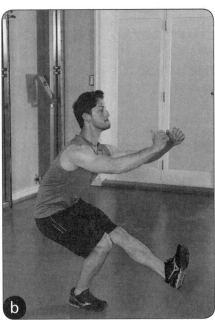

TRAINING TIP

This exercise is a true test of lower-body strength and stability! It is one of the top sport strength and conditioning exercises to build powerful leg muscles and joints. Get as deep as you can and use the chair behind you for support if needed. Challenge yourself to get a little deeper each week.

ONE-LEG-UP CRUNCHES

EXERCISE NOTES

- This is the third exercise in Hardcore Body-Weight Training Workout.
- Complete this exercise directly after performing one-leg pistol squats.
- Because this is the third exercise in your tri-set, you will rest after completing it.

Start

Step 1: Lie on your back and look directly up to the ceiling throughout the set.

Step 2: Lift one leg up at a right angle and keep the other leg out straight. Hold the leg that is out straight about 2 inches (5 cm) off the floor and have your knee extended straight.

Step 3: Place both hands to the sides of your head and keep your chin away from your chest.

Step 4: *(a)* Lift your upper back and head off the floor so that you can keep constant tension on your abdominal muscles throughout the set.

Midpoint

Step 5: *(b)* Crunch your chest toward the knee that is held up at a right angle but do not move your legs.

Step 6: Slowly lower your upper body back to the starting position but do not let your abs lose tension.

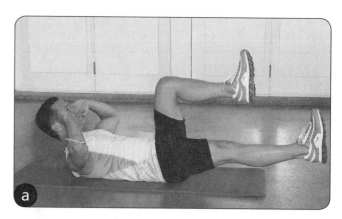

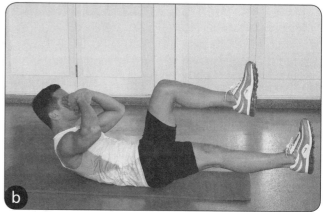

Finish

Step 7: Perform 10 to 15 reps with one leg up and then switch to the opposite side without letting your feet touch the ground or losing tension on your abs. Aim to get the same number of reps on each side and then rest.

TRAINING TIP

This exercise is deceptively difficult. Most guys think that they can just bang out 20 reps on each side, but if you're keeping constant tension on your abs you'll feel them burn up pretty quickly. The other good thing is that there isn't a lot of spinal flexion in this exercise, so it's a great exercise for those without lower back pain to make their abs stronger and more defined!

SIDE PLANKS WITH REACH UNDER

EXERCISE NOTES

- Complete the entire first tri-set two or three times before moving on to the second group of exercises.
- This is the first exercise in the second tri-set of Hardcore Body-Weight Training Workout.

Start

Step 1: Lie on your right side and place your right elbow directly below your right shoulder. Your right forearm should lie on the floor perpendicular to your body.

Step 2: Stack your left foot on top of your right foot and place your left arm straight up in the air so that it forms a 180-degree line with your right arm below.

Step 3: *(a)* Now push your hips off the floor so that only your right forearm and right foot and ankle are in contact with the floor.

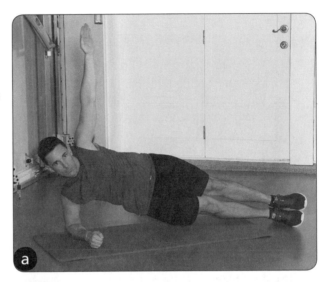

Midpoint

Step 4: *(b)* While maintaining your high hip position take the top (left) arm and reach under and around your body until you touch your right oblique or lower back area with your left palm.

Finish

Step 5: Bring your left arm back around your body and raise it back up straight in the air into its starting position.

Step 6: Repeat for the desired number of reps and then switch sides.

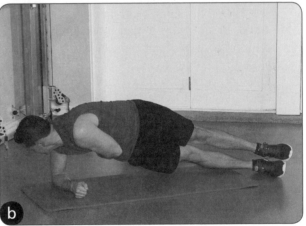

TRAINING TIP

The trick to completing this exercise properly is to keep your ear, shoulder, hip, knee, and ankle all lined up perfectly straight when you are maintaining your static side plank position. This positioning will engage your body in its proper kinetic chain, allow you to complete the movement using the correct muscles groups, and strengthen your core to a greater degree.

BULGARIAN SPLIT SQUATS WITH TWO-ARM RAISE

EXERCISE NOTES

- This is the second exercise in the second tri-set of Hardcore Body-Weight Training Workout.
- Complete this exercise directly after performing side planks with reach under.

Start

Step 1: Place a box or bench that is approximately knee height on the floor behind you.

Step 2: Place your hands by your sides and use your core to keep your chest up and spine in alignment.

Step 3: *(a)* Stand about 3 feet (90 cm) away from the bench and place the top of your right foot on the bench so that your ankle has room to move. You should now be standing on just your left foot.

Midpoint

Step 4: *(b)* Keeping the weight on your left heel and hip, sit back into those areas as you squat or lunge down until your back knee stretches down to just above the floor (your legs should resemble close to right angles at this point). As you are lowering your body down to the floor, simultaneously raise your arms above your shoulders.

Finish

Step 5: Push up through your left hip and heel as you stand back up to the starting position, still balancing on just your left leg.

Step 6: Repeat all reps on your left leg and then switch sides.

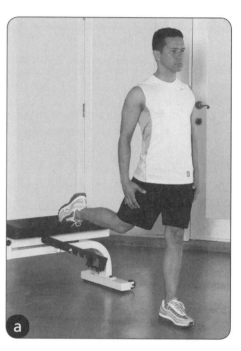

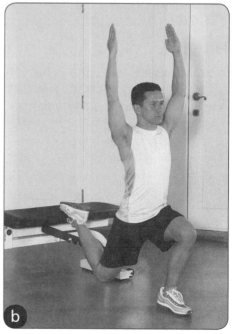

TRAINING TIP

Bulgarian split squats are really a lunge-based movement and target muscles similar to those targeted by a lunge. You should feel a stretch down the quadriceps and hip flexors of the leg that is on the bench, but the front leg should be the one working to take the weight. Allow the back leg to take little weight and instead use it just to keep you balanced.

ALTERNATING SUPERMANS

EXERCISE NOTES

- This is the third exercise in the second tri-set of Hardcore Body-Weight Training Workout.
- Complete this exercise directly after performing Bulgarian split squats with two-arm raise.
- Because this is the third exercise in your tri-set, you will rest after completing it.

Start

Step 1: Lie flat on your belly on a mat.

Step 2: Stretch out both your arms and your legs.

Step 3: *(a)* Looking straight down at the ground lift both arms and legs off the ground to begin to place tension on your posterior chain (the muscles on your back side).

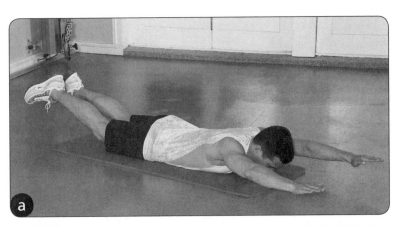

Midpoint

Step 4: *(b)* Squeeze your glutes and lift your left leg (including your quads) as far off the ground as you can while squeezing your upper back at the same time to lift your right arm. Do not pull your head up; keep looking at the floor below you.

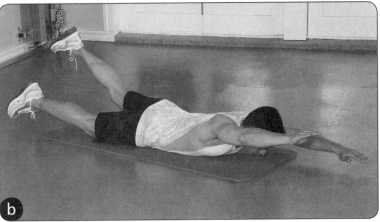

Finish

Step 5: Still keeping your right arm and left leg lifted high and fully extended, begin to lower those limbs down in a controlled manner to the starting position above the floor.

Step 6: Now lift your right leg and left arm in the same fashion. Continue alternating sides.

TRAINING TIP

I see many people move super fast through this exercise using momentum instead of muscle to complete each rep. Don't be that guy; it will hurt your back in the long run and will not help to strengthen weak posterior-chain muscles. Complete each rep deliberately and slowly to get the most out of each set. Don't worry about doing fewer reps until you become stronger. You will be far better off in the long run!

INCHWORMS

EXERCISE NOTES

- Complete the dynamic warm-up exercises first.
- This is the first exercise in the second workout of Hardcore Body-Weight Training Workout.

Start

Step 1: Stand with your legs together.

Step 2: *(a)* Place both hands directly on the floor in front of your feet.

Step 3: Keep your fingers and palms in contact with the ground throughout the set and begin walking your hands out, one after the other.

Midpoint

Step 4: *(b)* Make sure to keep your core engaged throughout the set so that your hips don't drop toward the floor. Walk your hands out past the push-up position if possible and stay on the balls of your feet.

Step 5: After you have walked your hands out as far as you can, begin to make small steps with your legs to walk your feet into your hands. Try to keep your knees straight and walk in only as far as your lower back and hamstrings will allow.

Finish

Step 6: After you have walked your feet in as far as you can to your hands, begin to walk your hands back out as far as you can and repeat the process. When you do the exercise correctly you will be walking your hands out and then walking your feet in with each rep to move forward down the floor.

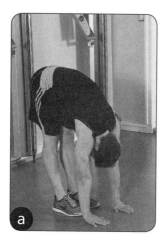 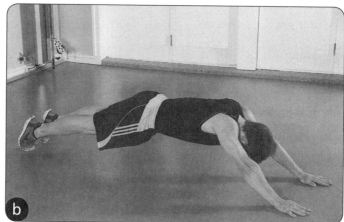

TRAINING TIP

Besides giving your backside a great stretch you work your shoulders and core with this fantastic movement. Remember to keep your fingers and palms in contact with the ground throughout the movement. Also, if you are working out in a small space you can tweak this exercise by walking your hands out, walking your feet in, walking your feet back out, and then walking your hands back to your feet. Repeat the pattern by walking your hands back out again.

ALTERNATING DYNAMIC FORWARD LUNGES

EXERCISE NOTES

- This is the second exercise in Hardcore Body-Weight Training Workout.
- Complete this exercise directly after performing inchworms.

Start

Step 1: *(a)* Stand with your feet slightly apart and hands at your sides.

Step 2: Step forward with your left leg while keeping the weight on the front heel and sitting into the front left hip.

Midpoint

Step 3: *(b)* Allow your back (right) knee to bend straight down to the ground and stop a few inches (8 or 10 cm) before touching the floor, while raising your arms into the air.

Finish

Step 4: Push through your left heel while raising your arms overhead back to the original starting position.

Step 5: Alternate sides with each repetition.

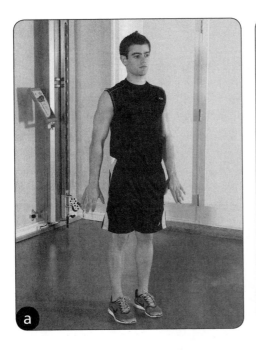 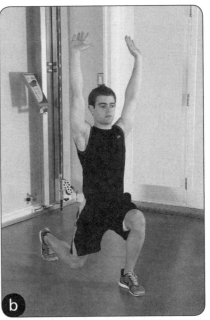

TRAINING TIP

Do not allow your weight to shift onto the ball of the front foot or let your front knee go over your toes. You should sit into the lunge by placing the weight on your front hip and heel.

CHAIR DIPS

EXERCISE NOTES

- This is the third exercise in Hardcore Body-Weight Training Workout.
- Complete this exercise directly after performing alternating dynamic forward lunges.
- Because this is the third exercise in your tri-set, you will rest after completing it.

Start

Step 1: Place a sturdy chair behind you.

Step 2: *(a)* Hold the edge of the chair so that your palms are facing away from you and walk your feet out so that your legs are straight.

Step 3: Keeping your elbows in alignment with your shoulders (do not allow them to flare out), slowly lower your hips toward the floor.

Midpoint

Step 4: *(b)* Stop when your biceps are parallel to the ground or just above that point if you are feeling unstable or tight through your shoulders.

Finish

Step 5: Squeeze your triceps and push yourself back to the starting position.

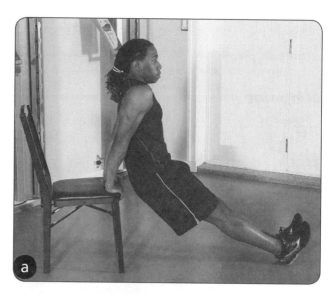

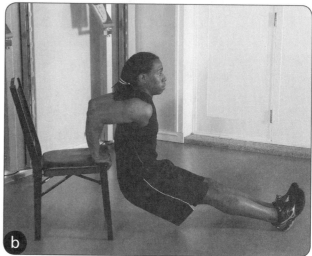

TRAINING TIP

I'm a huge fan of dips for triceps, shoulder, and chest development, but you must be careful to keep tension on those muscles all the way through the movement. Be sure not to stretch too deep and cause too much shoulder flexion. Also, because chair dips are typically a little easier then parallel bar dips, you can elevate your feet if you want to make this movement a little more challenging.

PLANKS WITH SHOULDER ABDUCTION

EXERCISE NOTES

- Complete the entire first tri-set two or three times before moving on to the second group of exercises.
- This is the first exercise in the second tri-set of Hardcore Body-Weight Training Workout.

Start

Step 1: *(a)* Lie on a mat in a plank position, have your forearms parallel to each other, and position your shoulders directly above your elbows.

Step 2: Keep your feet a maximum of hip-width apart.

Midpoint

Step 3: *(b)* Use the muscles behind your left shoulder to rotate or abduct your arm externally up at the same right angle that it currently has on the mat. When finished you should be looking down at the mat with your entire body still in a plank and only your left arm rotated out by your side at a right angle.

Finish

Step 4: Slowly lower your left arm back to the mat and place it in its starting position on your forearm.

Step 5: Repeat on your right side and continue alternating reps.

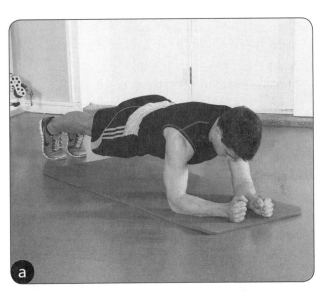

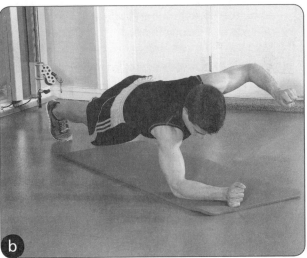

TRAINING TIP

This exercise is a great core challenge that really fires up your obliques and postural muscles! Concentrate on keeping your balance and not letting your hips drop down toward the floor as you rotate. Because we're trying to make this movement a little tougher, I suggest trying to keep your feet together after you master your balance. Good luck!

SHIN SLAP V-UPS

EXERCISE NOTES

- This is the second exercise in the second tri-set of Hardcore Body-Weight Training Workout.
- Complete this exercise directly after performing planks with shoulder abduction.

Start

Step 1: Lie on your back on a mat.

Step 2: Stretch both legs and both arms out straight.

Step 3: *(a)* Raise both arms, both legs, your upper back, and your head off the floor about 1 inch (2.5 cm) to keep tension on your abs.

Midpoint

Step 4: *(b)* Quickly raise both legs straight up in the air at the same time that you're lifting your arms overhead to meet your legs (they should intersect above your hips or just slightly toward your legs). As you're reaching this peak position you should literally slap your shins with both palms.

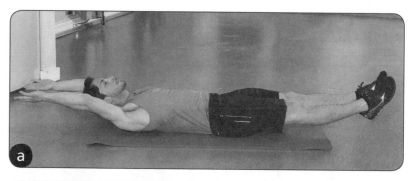

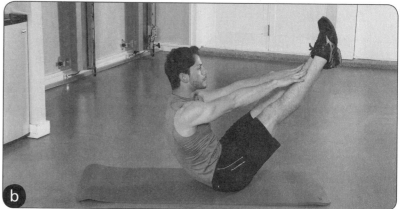

Step 5: After pausing for a second to squeeze and flex your abs, slowly lower both your upper body and your lower body back to the starting position (do not bend your elbows or knees at any point during this exercise).

Finish

Step 6: When you're about to lose tension on your abs or you've reached the starting position, go right into your next rep.

Step 7: Repeat for as many reps as possible with good form.

TRAINING TIP

This deceptively difficult exercise really pushes your abdominal and core strength to the limit. In addition, the harder you slap your shins, the more force you drive back into your core, making your abs work even harder! Just make sure not to round out your neck or back, and you'll enjoy all the benefits that this exercise has to offer.

ONE-LEG DYNAMIC BRIDGING

EXERCISE NOTES

- This is the third exercise in the second tri-set of Hardcore Body-Weight Training Workout.
- Complete this exercise directly after performing shin slap V-ups.
- Because this is the third exercise in your tri-set, you will rest after completing it.

Start

Step 1: Lie on your back.

Step 2: Pull both feet into your hips.

Step 3: Fold your arms across your chest.

Step 4: Keep your knees directly over your ankles and then lift your right leg off the mat and hold it up in the air throughout the movement.

Step 5: Engage your glutes by squeezing them together.

Midpoint

Step 6: *(a)* Keeping your glutes engaged, exhale and push your hips off the mat as high as you can lift them without lifting your left heel.

Finish

Step 7: *(b)* Slowly breathe in and lower your hips to 1 inch (2.5 cm) above the mat (do not touch the mat).

Step 8: Repeat by lifting and lowering your hips slowly.

Step 9: After completing 12 to 15 repetitions with your left side, place your right foot back down on the floor and lift your left leg up in the air to work your right side.

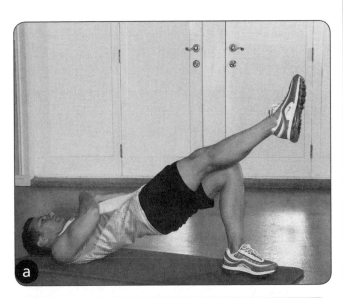

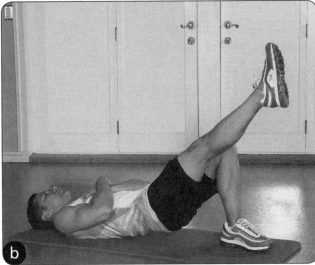

TRAINING TIP

Stay focused on using your glutes throughout the movement by squeezing them forcefully on the way up and making sure that they stay level to the floor. If your hamstrings cramp up, it is a sure sign that they are overactive and that your glutes aren't working hard enough!

HINDU PUSH-UPS

EXERCISE NOTES

- Complete the dynamic warm-up exercises first.
- This is the first exercise in the third workout of Hardcore Body-Weight Training Workout.
- This workout is circuit based, so you will complete all five exercises in a row without resting.
- After you complete all five exercises you can rest for two or three minutes before repeating the circuit.

Start

Step 1: Get into push-up position on the floor.

Step 2: *(a)* Lift your hips high up into the air so that you sit back into your legs, stretching your lower back, glutes, hamstrings, and calves. Your body should resemble an upside-down V (think of this as the downward-facing dog pose in yoga).

Step 3: Next, dive bomb down with your head and upper body toward the floor, keeping your elbows in close to your body. I like to think of this as running my nose along the floor before lifting up.

Midpoint

Step 4: *(b)* Lift your upper body and head up into the air as you raise your chest high. At this point your hips should be about 1 inch (2.5 cm) off the floor, and you should be squeezing your glutes and triceps (resembles the upward-facing dog pose in yoga).

Finish

Step 5: Drop your head down toward the floor and shift your hips back to the starting position so that they are raised high into the air stretching your posterior chain.

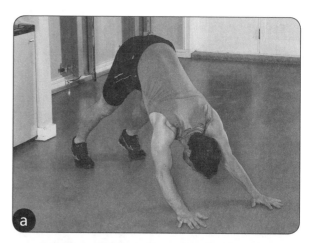

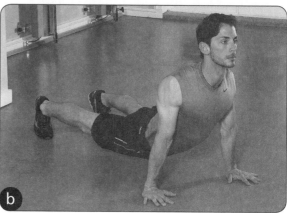

TRAINING TIP

This exercise may seem complex at first, but it is meant to flow from one rep to the next as in the downward- and upward-facing dog poses from yoga. It's a great exercise at stretching not only your upper body but also your tight leg and hip muscles. With a little practice you'll master the form in no time!

PRISONER DEEP SQUATS

EXERCISE NOTES

- This is the second exercise in the Hardcore Body-Weight Training Workout.
- Complete this exercise directly after performing Hindu push-ups.

Start

Step 1: Place a flat 12-inch (30 cm) box or object behind you as you stand with your feet hip-width apart and your knees slightly bent.

Step 2: Maintain a flat back (neutral spine) and retract your shoulder blades for posture throughout the set. Also, make sure to keep your chest up and your chin parallel to the floor.

Step 3: *(a)* Clasp your hands behind your head (prisoner position) and keep them locked in place throughout the set.

Midpoint

Step 4: Slowly breathe in and sit back with your hips into a full deep squat, keeping the weight on your heels.

Step 5: *(b)* Get as deep as you can (using the box to practice form if needed) without excessively rounding out your lower back, letting your heels come up, dropping your chest, or going into a posterior pelvic tilt.

Finish

Step 6: Push as hard you can through your hips and heels to propel yourself back to the standing start position.

Step 7: Exhale on the way up and repeat your next repetition when ready.

TRAINING TIP

These body-weight prisoner deep squats are fantastic for strengthening your legs at a position deeper then you would go with a barbell on your shoulders or a pair of dumbbells in your hands. You'll begin to feel more powerful and comfortable in this deep position, which will lead to better results when you get back to hitting the weights!

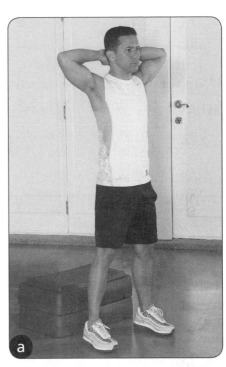

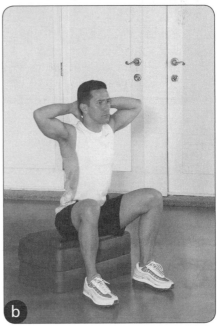

BRAZILIAN CRUNCHES

EXERCISE NOTES

- This is the third exercise in the third workout of Hardcore Body-Weight Training Workout.
- Complete this exercise directly after performing prisoner deep squats.

Start

Step 1: *(a)* Get into a push-up position on the floor and keep your shoulders directly over your wrists throughout the set.

Step 2: Keep your core engaged and do not let your hips sag down or lift too high in the air.

Midpoint

Step 3: *(b)* Lift your left leg off the ground and bring that knee under your chest to the opposite right elbow. Try to touch the knee to right above the opposite elbow.

Finish

Step 4: Next, lift your right leg off the floor and try to touch just above your left elbow with it.

Step 5: Repeat by alternating sides with each rep.

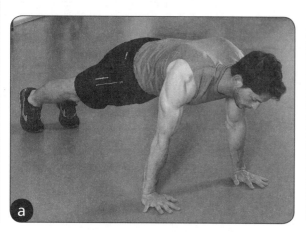 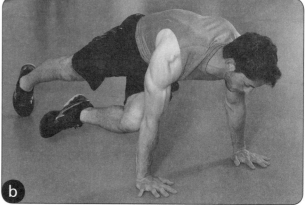

TRAINING TIP

This hardcore abdominal and oblique movement works the entire core. My tip to get the most out of this exercise is to stretch your hips as much as possible while flexing your abs so that you can get your knee to touch above the opposite elbow. Just make sure not to drop your hips as you go to crunch in with your knee.

ONE-LEG GOOD MORNINGS

EXERCISE NOTES

- This is the fourth exercise in the third workout of Hardcore Body-Weight Training Workout.
- Complete this exercise directly after performing Brazilian crunches.

Start

Step 1: Stand with your feet hip-width apart and your knees slightly bent.

Step 2: Cross your arms over your chest.

Step 3: Maintain a flat back (neutral spine) and retract your shoulder blades for posture throughout the set. Also, make sure to keep your chest up and core engaged.

Midpoint

Step 4: *(a)* Slowly breathe in and sit back with your hips, keeping the weight on your heels as you lift your right leg off the ground and kick straight back with it.

Step 5: *(b)* Stretch as deep you can into your left hip and hamstring while allowing your back to lower slowly toward the floor.

Finish

Step 6: Push through your hips and lift your upper body back up to standing position, squeezing the left glute area and not allowing the right foot to touch if possible (or just tap the ball of the right foot as you come to the top).

Step 7: Repeat all repetitions on one side before switching sides.

TRAINING TIP

The one-leg good morning is a powerful exercise that will really test your balance. Concentrate on each rep and never stretch past the point of tension or round out your lower back at any point during the set.

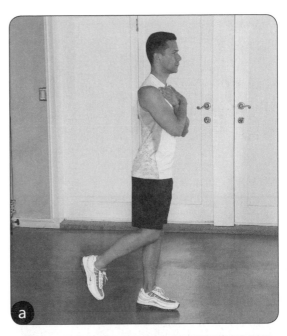

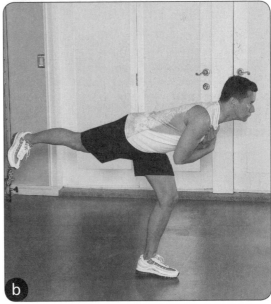

SQUAT THRUSTS (BURPEES)

EXERCISE NOTES

- Complete this exercise after performing one-leg good mornings.
- This is the fifth exercise in the third workout of Hardcore Body-Weight Training Workout.
- Because this is the final exercise of the circuit, you will rest two or three minutes after completing it before beginning the five-exercise circuit again.

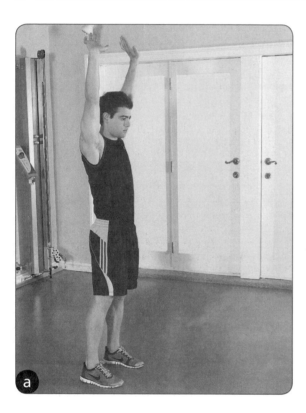 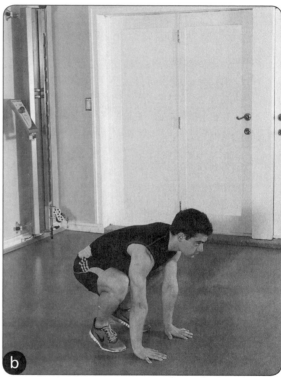

Start

Step 1: *(a)* Stand with your feet hip-width apart and your arms raised overhead.

Step 2: *(b)* Bend over and place your hands on the floor about shoulder-width apart in front of your feet.

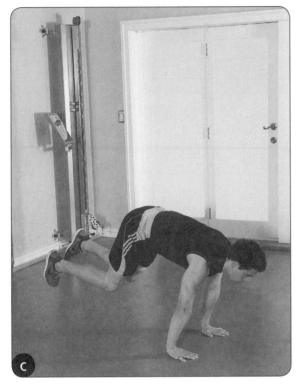

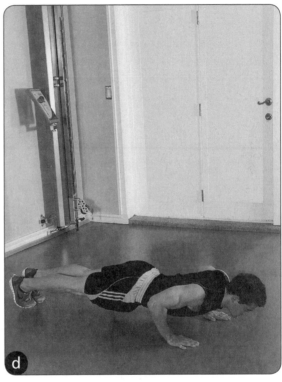

Midpoint

Step 3: (c) Jump back with both legs and land in a push-up position (engage your core and do not let your hips sag down toward the floor).

Step 4: (d) Complete a push-up.

Finish

Step 5: From the top of your push-up, jump both legs back up to your hands.

Step 6: Stand back up straight and raise your arms over your head.

Step 7: Repeat 10 times as fast as you can with good form.

TRAINING TIP

If you are concerned about your form or joints when you are asked to jump back and jump in, I recommend placing one foot back (or in) at a time to minimize the force on your joints. Concentrate on landing softly and absorbing the impact.

CHAPTER 14

The Road Ahead

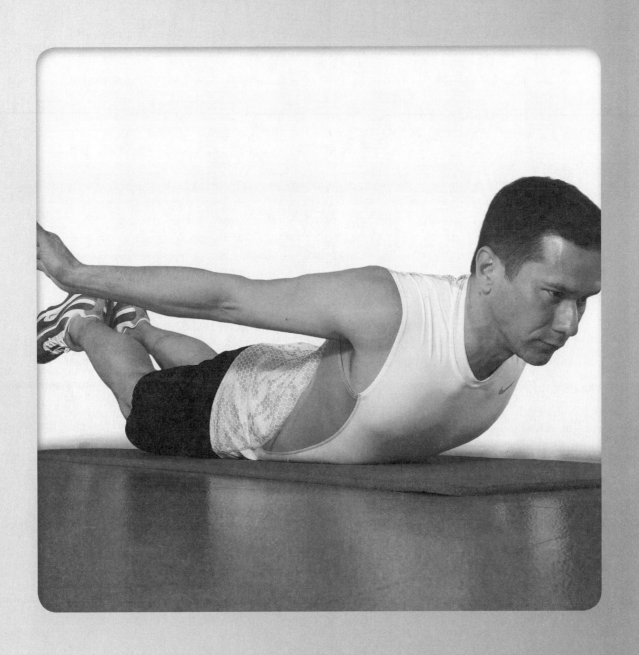

What to do now . . .

By the time you get to this chapter you may have already completed a few or all of the men's strength and conditioning training programs that I wrote specifically for you. And if you did, you noticed that an entire year's worth of workouts is loaded into this workout manual. Of course, after completing the starter programs you're welcome to skip around and choose the workout that best suits your needs at this time in your life.

Eventually, however, you will have worked through every program and mastered all the lifts. At that point you have two choices:

1. You can go back where you started and begin the programs again, only this time try to increase your weights now that you have another year of lifting under your belt. (That is why you should write your weights and reps into the tables that I provided for you.)

2. You can visit reputable websites for new and updated workouts, articles, and everything related to health and fitness.

Another point I want to make is that after seriously training with these powerful workouts, you will have a deeper level of training knowledge that you can put to good use for the rest of your life. You should be able to pick out poorly designed and imbalanced workouts, and avoid exercises that are unsafe or will only hinder your progress. Remember, it's all about growth. Not only are your muscles growing, but you're growing as a man as well.

Committing to a strength and conditioning program sets you apart from the 9 out of 10 guys who just can't be bothered. They've given up on themselves and their bodies. They've decided that the effort isn't worth it. Boy, are they wrong.

A lifetime of strength training has been shown to keep you leaner, stronger, and younger when compared with men your age who choose not to be physically active. In addition, every time you lift, surges of testosterone and other beneficial hormones race through your body, making you feel great, both physically and mentally.

For myself, and many other guys, strength training is a way to enjoy some "me time" and get away from work, commitments, and other stresses that tug at you all day long. Even if it's only for 20 to 30 minutes a few times per week, a solid workout can rejuvenate you from the inside out. That is why I urge you never to stop what you have started.

Between proper nutrition, healthy lifestyle maintenance, and this powerful strength-training manual, you hold the keys to success. Use them. Share what you've learned with others.

Together, we can positively change the sedentary culture that surrounds us. You need to participate in the change that you want to see in the world, and to be a positive role model for others you need to practice what you preach. So, of course, do it for yourself—train to get stronger, more fit, more athletic, leaner, more defined, and more powerful—but at the same time share your experience with others.

I truly hope that you enjoyed actively using this men's strength-training guide. I had a blast designing it and laying out everything in a way that I thought would help you learn best. One day I look forward to hearing your success stories.

Enjoy the road the ahead.

References

Aaberg, Everett. 2006. *Muscle Mechanics, 2nd Edition*. Champaign: Human Kinetics.

Aaberg, Everett. 1999. *Resistance Training Instruction*. Champaign: Human Kinetics.

Baechle, Thomas R. and Roger W. Earle. 2008. *Essentials of Strength Training and Conditioning, 3rd Edition*. Champaign: Human Kinetics.

Calorie Burn Calculator by Health Status. http://www.healthstatus.com/calculate/cbc

Koch, Richard. 1999. "The 80/20 Principle: The Secret to Achieving More with Less." *Crown Business*. 19 October.

Kang, J., N. Ratamess, A. Faigenbaum, and J. Hoffman. 2003. "EPOC, Human Performance Lab." *Journal of Applied Physiology and Occupational Physiology*.

Poliquin, Charles. 1994. *German Body Comp Program*. Phoenix: Poliquin Performance Center.

Staley, Charles. 2005. *Muscle Logic: Escalating Density Training*. New York: Rodale Books.

Tabata, I., K. Nishimura, M. Kouzaki, et al. 1996. "Effects of moderate-intensity endurance and high-intensity intermittent training on anaerobic capacity and $\dot{V}O_2$max." *Med Sci Sports Exerc*. 28 (10): 1327-30.

About the Author

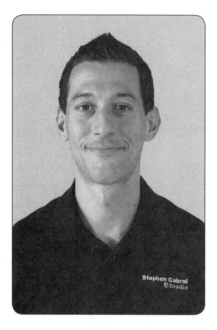

Stephen Cabral was voted the 2011 PFP Personal Trainer of the Year and has completed more than 15,000 private training sessions since 1999, helping athletes, CEOs, doctors, stay-at-home moms, and everyone in between reach their goals. He specializes in breaking down seemingly complex concepts into bite-sized chunks of information that people can digest and put to use. Cabral takes great pride in changing people's lives by changing their bodies.

As the resident health and fitness expert for NutritionData, Gather.com, Self.com, Diet.com, and a host of other companies looking to inspire their members through proper strength training and weight loss, Cabral has written and published over 1,100 articles. He has also appeared as a celebrity trainer on the reality TV show *Survival of the Richest* and worked with MTV's *Made* for six weeks as a strength training expert helping a contestant get into shape the fastest way possible.

In addition to his writing and training network, Stephen Cabral has shot more than 100 fitness videos that have been seen by well over 3 million viewers online. "The Best Ab Exercises You've Never Heard Of" generated over a million views alone. His partnership with Diet.com, meanwhile, has enabled the site to produce numerous high-quality, award-winning videos for YouTube, including one that was voted the top how-to video out of hundreds of thousands of competitors.

The personal newsletter that Cabral writes is read by more than 100,000 people each week at www.StephenCabral.com.